T0250168

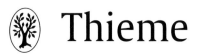

This book is dedicated to
Leena Lalitha and Vedanth Daneel

An Illustrated Handbook of Flap-Raising Techniques

Kartik G. Krishnan, MD

Department of Neurosurgery
Carl Gustav Carus University Hospital
Dresden, Germany

110 illustrations

Georg Thieme Verlag
Stuttgart · New York

Library of Congress Cataloging-in-Publication Data
Krishnan, Kartik G.
An illustrated handbook of flap-raising techniques /
Kartik G. Krishnan.
p. ; cm.
Includes bibliographical references.
ISBN 978-3-13-147761-3 (alk. paper)
1. Flaps (Surgery)–Handbooks, manuals, etc. I. Title.
[DNLM: 1. Surgical Flaps–Handbooks. 2. Microsurgery–
methods–Handbooks. 3. Reconstructive Surgical
Procedures–methods–Handbooks. WO 39 K92i 2008]
RD120.8.K75 2008
617.9'5–dc22

© 2008 Georg Thieme Verlag,
Rüdigerstrasse 14, 70469 Stuttgart, Germany
http://www.thieme.de
Thieme New York, 333 Seventh Avenue,
New York, NY 10001, USA
http://www.thieme.com

Cover design: Thieme Publishing Group
Typesetting by Mitterweger & Partner, Plankstadt
Printed in Germany by Graphisches Centrum Cuno
GmbH, Calbe
ISBN987-3-13-147761-3

1 2 3 4 5 6

Preface

Since the development of microsurgical techniques and discovery of consistently repeated vascular patterns of tissues, the face of reconstructive surgery, or rather the face of surgery as a whole, has totally changed. Any established training program in plastic and reconstructive surgery devotes, in parallel to clinical work, a considerable amount of time to revisiting specific nuances in the anatomy laboratory, as well as to mastering microsurgical techniques, both being integrated fundaments, upon which the practice of plastic surgery is built. Anatomical dissections for learning specific surgical techniques, especially as pertinent to the harvesting of flaps, are best accomplished by referring to a written and illustrated resource kept readily open on a book rack there and then, as one proceeds with the dissection.

A textbook is a tool with an intentional purpose and utility. Even when covering the same topic, two books may have a completely different scope and focus. There are a variety of excellent written resources on reconstructive surgery using flaps, which compete and complement each other as regards the fundus of scientific material they command. Depending upon the requirements of the reader, one resource may be of great value, while another may be of little interest.

Here I would like to impart some of my experience as a trainee in plastic and reconstructive surgery: on-call-free Saturdays were an excellent time in the anatomy laboratory for learning the harvesting of flaps. Before I went on these missions, considerable homework was required; I used to refer to various volumes on reconstructive surgery, cull the most relevant information as pertinent to the anatomical nuances and surgical technique of the flaps I had planned to harvest the next day, and make appropriate sketches and scribble essential notes that I would take with me to the laboratory. This discipline accompanied me further into the operating room while doing clinical work, and continues to do so when attending to challenging cases.

The discovery and improvisation of surgical flaps have developed via a painstaking route of enormous effort in innovative thinking, and meticulous search for the lurking truths, adding steadily to the volumes of existing literature. The result of such consistent scientific endeavors is seen in today's practice of surgery. However, when one is confronted with the question of "how to do it," the historical nuances of scientific discovery disappear into the background and serve as a strong basis, upon which the variations of techniques are held.

This manual, *An Illustrated Handbook of Flap Raising Techniques*, is in no way unique. As already mentioned, there are already volumes devoted to the topic. This presentation is a compilation of my schematic diagrams and sketches, notes on the technical nuances, and observations on the pitfalls, which I found most useful during the phase of my learning to harvest free flaps. Nor does this manual claim to preach wisdom, rather it hopes to accompany the user toward it, by means of aiding him or her in persistent technical accomplishments. Bearing these qualities in mind, the text and literature references are kept to a minimum, with more offerings of diagrammatic sequences to assist in understanding by viewing the illustrations. There are numerous flaps that were not treated in this selection; flaps of the hand, head and neck, and perforator flaps for example. The manual concentrates, rather, on the most versatile flaps that are quickly learned and easy to harvest.

This handbook claims to be a technical companion for flap surgery, but its aim would not be substantiated without mention of microvascular and microneural sutures. Two chapters at the end of the manual are devoted to techniques in microsurgery, which might be considered useful as an introduction into these areas. I only hope that this collection of artwork and corresponding description is brief enough to be quickly covered, and at the same time elaborate enough to provide an impetus for furthering the search, to have created a book that will benefit the reader.

Kartik G. Krishnan, MD

Acknowledgements

I would like to acknowledge many individuals who have, directly or indirectly, made this manual possible. The project was initially discussed with Dr. Clifford Bergman at Thieme Publishers, Stuttgart. I would like to thank the staff at Thieme Publishers for their help in producing this manual.

I also wish to thank the influence of my teachers and mentors who imparted their knowledge and provided leadership by example. In particular, Professor Vladislav Kulikov from the Department of Normal Human Anatomy at the Russian State Medical University, Moscow—a great thinker who encouraged my enquiry into *materia anatomica* when I was a medical student. Drs. Vsevolod V. Rybchonok and Alexander Razumovsky created an atmosphere of academic excellence as professors of plastic and reconstructive microsurgery and pediatric surgery, respectively, during my pursuit of plastic surgery. But for the striking example and mentorship of these two surgeons, I would not be the surgeon I am today. Professor Leonhard Schweiberer, former director of the surgical clinics of Ludwig Maximilian University in Munich and Professor Wolfgang Stock, Head of the Department of Plastic Surgery at the same institution, developed an infrastructure conducive to academic pursuit and wholeheartedly supported my interest in reconstructive surgery and associated research.

During my further training in neurological surgery, a number of individuals have served to accompany me in my development, and at the same time encouraged me to integrate plastic surgical principles into neurosurgical practice: Professor Peter A. Winkler and Professor Hans-Juergen Reulen at the Department of Neurosurgery, Ludwig Maximilian University Munich introduced me to neurosurgical thinking, without compromising plastic surgical ways. Professor Gabriele Schackert from the Department of Neurosurgery at Carl Gustav Carus University Hospital was a guiding light thoroughout the phase of my metamorphosis into a fully-fledged neurosurgeon and encouraged me to pursue academic activities in neurosurgery.

I would like to acknowledge the students, residents, and visiting fellows with whom I became acquainted on the undergraduate and postgraduate training programs at the Carl Gustav Carus University Hospital. Many of the sketches in this book have grown from teaching presentations made for trainees. I am most grateful to the physicians of Saxony and the surgeons at the Carl Gustav Carus University Hospital, who have referred many of their patients over the years, thus enabling me to broaden my experience.

Upon my request, Anna Krishnan kindly painted the movement studies on the section openers, for which I am thankful.

Finally I am grateful for the support of my parents, Lalitha and Gopal of Madras, India, who years ago provided a home environment where questions could be asked, the acquisition of new knowledge was encouraged, and scholarly pursuits were nurtured.

Table of Contents

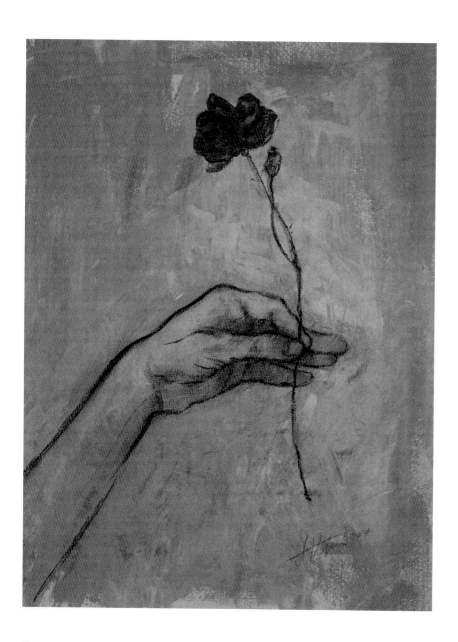

Part 1
Flaps of the Upper Extremity

Part 1
Flaps of the Upper Extremity

The upper extremity offers a variety of flaps to be raised either as free microvascular flaps (e.g., forearm flaps, lateral arm flap), or as pedicled flaps for reconstruction of defects in the anatomical neighborhood (e.g., distally pedicled flaps of the forearm for hand reconstruction).

Several free muscle flaps of the upper extremity have been described in the literature, for example, free vascularized and innervated flexor digitorum superficialis muscle flap reported for motor reanimation in facial paralysis. In my opinion, these are a little too ambitious for the beginner, whom this manual addresses. Even among the small choice described here, the flaps demonstrate a variety of properties. For instance, the lateral arm flap is thin, relatively hairless, and offers sensory innervation, useful in hand reconstruction; the posterior interosseous flap is yet another thin skin flap, practically devoid of subcutaneous fat. These properties are favorably harnessed to meet specific reconstructive requirements.

The hand offers specific flaps for regional reconstruction: some examples are the pedicled V-Y flap based on the digital vessels and nerves, which is advanced and, if appropriate, rotated for finger tip reconstruction, and the Foucher flap from the dorsal 2nd metacarpal area for reconstruction of the thumb.

In this section, I have limited myself to the description of five flaps from the arm and forearm and some of their variations. As already mentioned, the upper extremity has much more to offer than these five. Mastery of the flaps described here will provide the practitioner with certain basics in flap manipulation, upon which he or she might be able to build skills that can ideally be extended to more challenging flaps.

Chapter 1
The Deltoid Fasciocutaneous Flap

The deltoid free flap is a neurovascular fasciocutaneous tissue, providing relatively thin sensate tissue for use in soft-tissue reconstruction. The deltoid fasciocutaneous flap was first described anatomically and applied clinically by Franklin.[1] Since then, the deltoid flap has been widely studied and applied.[2–5] This flap is supplied by a perforating branch of the posterior circumflex humeral artery and receives sensation by means of the lateral brachial cutaneous nerve and an inferior branch of the axillary nerve. This anatomy is a constant feature, thus making the flap reliable. The ideal free deltoid flap will be thin, hairless, of an adequate size, and capable of sensory reinnervation. These characteristics of the flap make it an attractive option for reconstructing defects of the orofacial region. However, in adipose individuals, the fat tissue might add to the bulk of the flap.

Preparation

The course of the neurovascular pedicle is determined and marked before surgery as follows. With the patient in sitting or standing position, the acromion and the lateral humeral epicondyle are palpated and marked. A straight line is marked to connect these two landmarks. The groove between the posterior border of the deltoid muscle and the long head of triceps is palpated and marked. The intersection of these two lines denotes approximately the location of the vascular pedicle, as it emerges from underneath the deltoid muscle. This point may be studied with a hand-held Doppler and marked if required.

Depending on the recipient area, the patient is positioned either supine, with the donor shoulder sufficiently padded with a stack of towels, or in the lateral decubitus position. Myorelaxants are required in muscular individuals, so as to ease retraction of the posterior border of the deltoid muscle, especially if a long vascular pedicle is required for reconstruction.

Neurovascular Anatomy

A large portion of the fasciocutaneous territory overlying the deltoid muscle is nourished by the posterior circumflex humeral artery with its paired venae comitantes (**Fig. 1.1**). The sensory innervation of this skin area is through the lateral brachial cutaneous nerve, which is the terminal sensory branch of the axillary nerve, a musculocutaneous nerve arising from the posterior cord. This nerve accompanies the vascular pedicle, passing behind the humerus and emerging from the quadrangular space, which is bordered by the teres major muscle below,

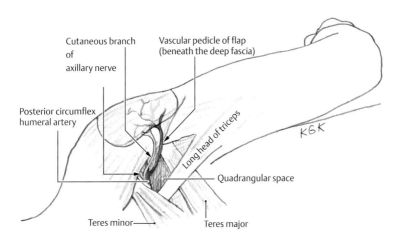

Cutaneous branch of axillary nerve

Vascular pedicle of flap (beneath the deep fascia)

Posterior circumflex humeral artery

Long head of triceps

Quadrangular space

Teres minor

Teres major

Fig. 1.1 Anatomical basis of the deltoid flap.

Fig. 1.2 Planning markings of the deltoid flap.

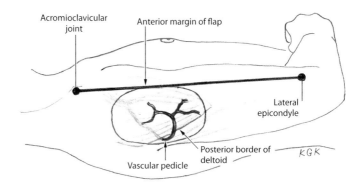

teres minor muscle above, long head of triceps medially, and the lateral head of triceps laterally. The vascular pedicle gives off branches to the deltoid muscles before its emergence. The nerve, as already mentioned, is a musculocutaneous nerve and provides motor innervation to the deltoid muscle. The neurovascular pedicle emerges at the posteroinferior border of the deltoid muscle, turns cranially after its emergence, and supplies the skin overlying the posterolateral aspect of the deltoid muscle. Thus a safe flap will be carved behind the line connecting the acromioclavicular joint and the lateral epicondyle, with an adducted and internally rotated arm (**Fig. 1.2**).

Incisions and Dissection

With the patient's arm adducted and internally rotated, three lines are drawn[1]: a line connecting the acromion and the lateral epicondyle,[2] a line along the groove between the posterior border of the deltoid muscle and the long head of triceps, and a line connecting the acromioc-

lavicular junction with lateral epicondyle.[3] The intersection of the first two lines denotes the point where the vascular pedicle emerges to the surface behind the deltoid muscle; whereas the third line should ideally be the anterior border of the planned skin flap. Any variation in the point of emergence of the vascular pedicle can be marked before surgery using a handheld Doppler.

The anterior border of the marked skin flap is incised first, extending it along the inferior border as required. The deep fascia overlying the deltoid muscle is sharply cut and the flap is elevated in a plane underneath the fascia. Dissection proceeds toward the vascular pedicle, which is visualized in the under surface of the flap, after partially raising it (**Fig. 1.3**). An occasional perforator from the deltoid muscle should be coagulated and divided. The neurovascular pedicle is traced to the delto-tricipital groove and carefully isolated. Now the rest of the skin incision can be completed (**Fig. 1.4**). The posterior border of the deltoid muscle is retracted to gain length of the vascu-

Fig. 1.3 Dissection of the deltoid flap.

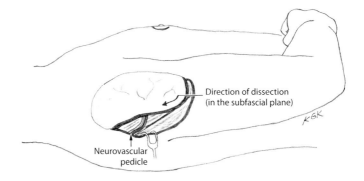

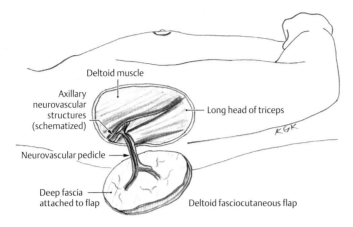

Fig. 1.4   Raising the deltoid flap.

Deltoid muscle

Axillary neurovascular structures (schematized)

Long head of triceps

Neurovascular pedicle

Deep fascia attached to flap

Deltoid fasciocutaneous flap

lar pedicle. Care should be taken to identify, isolate, and preserve nerves and vessels supplying the deltoid muscle.

Donor site closure is made by applying a meshed split-thickness skin graft. In cases where a vascularized fascia, and not the skin, is required (e.g., internal reconstruction, anterior skull base closure), the wound is closed on primary intention, after placing a suction drain in the dead space created by the harvested fascia.

The vascular pedicle is usually 6–8 cm long. The artery and the vein respectively have diameters of ~1.5–2 mm at the point of emergence from the delto-tricipital groove. Further proximal dissection of the vessels toward the posterior circumflex artery and veins will offer a diameter 1–2 mm larger. The neural pedicle is comparable in length to the vascular one.

> **Pitfalls**
>
> The length of the neurovascular pedicle is enhanced by following it in the depth behind the deltoid muscle. In doing so, it should be noted that the motor branches innervating the deltoid muscle should be carefully identified, isolated, and preserved. Failure to do so will result in paresis and rapid muscle atrophy.

There are cosmetic concerns in transplanting a split-skin mesh graft to the donor site, which cannot be avoided. It usually results in a contour depression of the donor area, preventing young female patients from wearing sleeveless shirts. These aspects need to be addressed in receiving informed consent before the flap is planned.

References

1   Franklin JD. The deltoid flap: anatomy and clinical applications. In: Buncke HJ, Furnas DW, eds. Symposium on Clinical Frontiers in Reconstructive Microsurgery. Vol. 24. St. Louis, Mo: Mosby; 1984

2   *Russell RC, Guy RJ, Zook EG, Merrell JC.* Extremity reconstruction using the free deltoid flap. Plast Reconstr Surg 1985;76:586–595

3   *Volpe CM, Peterson S, Doerr RJ, Karakousis CP.* Forequarter amputation with fasciocutaneous deltoid flap reconstruction for malignant tumors of the upper extremity. Ann Surg Oncol 1997;4:298–302

4   *Harashina T, Inoue T, Tanaka I, Imai K, Hatoko M.* Reconstruction of penis with free deltoid flap. Br J Plast Surg 1990;43:217–222

5   *Mathes SJ, Vasconez LO.* The cervico-humeral flap. Plast Reconstr Surg 1978;61:7–13

Chapter 2
The Lateral Arm Flap

The skin flap from the lateral arm region is based on the radial collateral artery arising from the profunda brachii artery and was first described by Song and colleagues in 1982.[1] The skin flap is thin, pliable, and relatively hairless, buttressing its use in facial reconstruction. Although being a thin flap in comparison to others, it may be found to be bulky when placing it over flap surfaces, as in hand reconstruction. It may be raised as a sensate as well as a composite flap along with a portion of the humeral shaft.[2,3] Anatomical studies in this decade have shown that the size of the free lateral arm flap may be safely extended into the forearm region.[4]

Preparation

The patient is positioned supine, with the donor upper extremity either spread on a hand table in a pronated position, as when hand reconstruction of the same extremity is called for, or internally rotated and adducted to the torso. A tourniquet is applied at the level of the proximal arm to ensure bloodless manipulation.

Neurovascular Anatomy

The posterior radial collateral artery, commonly named the radial collateral artery and the artery of the described flap, arises as a branch of the profunda brachii artery. The artery penetrates the lateral intermuscular septum distal to the deltoid insertion, and runs along the spiral groove lying in close proximity to the radial nerve, and continues distally toward the lateral epicondyle. Along its course, the artery gives off branches to periosteum, muscle, and skin (**Figs. 2.1, 2.2**). The periosteal branches supply the lower lateral aspect of the humerus in a segmental fashion. The artery gives off branches to the brachialis and brachioradialis muscles anteriorly and to the triceps muscle posteriorly, so that one of these tendons may be raised with a composite flap.

The posterior radial collateral artery runs along the lateral intermuscular septum of the arm and supplies the overlying skin through numerous tiny perforators. About 4–4.5 cm proximal to the lateral epicondyle, the main

Fig. 2.1 Anatomical basis of the lateral arm flap.

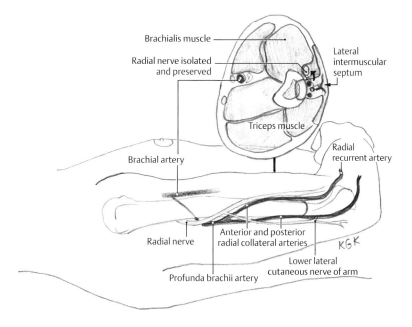

Brachialis muscle

Radial nerve isolated and preserved

Lateral intermuscular septum

Triceps muscle

Radial recurrent artery

Brachial artery

Radial nerve

Anterior and posterior radial collateral arteries

Lower lateral cutaneous nerve of arm

Profunda brachii artery

KGK

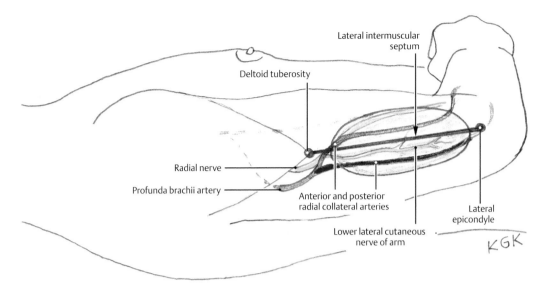

Lateral intermuscular
septum

Deltoid tuberosity

Radial nerve

Profunda brachii artery

Anterior and posterior
radial collateral arteries

Lateral
epicondyle

Lower lateral cutaneous
nerve of arm

KGK

Fig. 2.2   Planning markings of the lateral arm flap.

arterial trunk of the posterior radial collateral artery divides into its terminal branches and forms an expanded network. This network supplies the skin on the lateral aspect of the forearm. (**Fig. 2.1** is schematized; the vascular trunk shown here to be descending further distally to the epicondyle is not present in reality.)

At the elbow, the anterior as well as the posterior radial collateral arteries proceed posteriorly, taking a superficial course, to join the olecranon vascular network, which is fed additionally by the ulnar collateral arteries from proximally, and the radial and ulnar recurrent arteries from distally.

The lower lateral cutaneous nerve of the arm and the posterior cutaneous nerve of the forearm are sensory branches of the radial nerve that nourish the lower lateral aspect of the arm (the conventional lateral arm flap) and the posterolateral aspect of the forearm (the extended lateral arm flap), respectively. These nerves lie along the dissection path to the posterior radial collateral artery, the pedicle of the flap.

Incisions and Dissection

The insertion of the deltoid muscle and the lateral epicondyle of the humerus are palpated and marked. A straight line joining these points

marks the lateral intermuscular septum of the arm; this is where the posterior radial collateral artery lies. The flap is centered over this long axis and may be maximally 10 cm in width (**Fig. 2.2**). The length of the flap may be extended into the proximal forearm.

The posterior skin incision, reaching till the deep fascia, is made first. Then the dissection is performed from distal to proximal in the subfascial plane. One sees vascular ramifications of the radial collateral arteries superficial to the translucent deep fascia as the dissection proceeds. Both posterior and anterior radial collateral arteries are identified a little distally to the insertion of the deltoid muscle. Accompanying the posterior radial collateral artery is the lower lateral cutaneous nerve of the arm and, more distally, the posterior cutaneous nerve of the forearm, both arising from the radial nerve. Following the collateral arteries more proximally brings us to the profunda brachii artery that lies along with the radial nerve in the spiral groove (**Fig. 2.3**). It is important to respect this nerve and isolate it from possible injuries while raising the flap. Having identified the neurovascular structures of the flap, the anterior skin incision is made and dissection is performed in the subfascial plane above the bellies of the brachialis and brachioradialis muscles (**Fig. 2.4**).

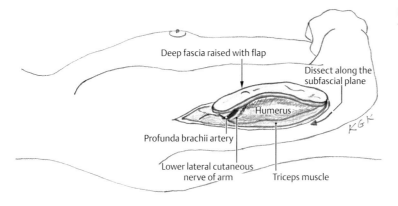

Fig. 2.3 Dissection of the lateral arm flap.

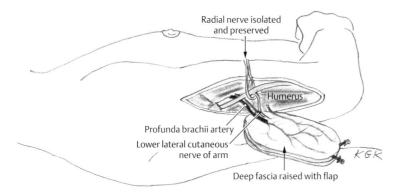

Fig. 2.4 Raising the lateral arm flap.

The pedicle length is ~5–6 cm; a further 1–1.5 cm extension is possible by carefully dissecting into the spiral groove. Vessel diameters are usually 1–1.5 mm.

The dissection technique of the osteoseptocutaneous lateral arm flap is a little different. After making the posterior incision, the flap is raised in the subfascial plane toward the marked long axis. The lateral intermuscular septum is identified at a distal point of the flap. Then dissection proceeds into the matter of the triceps muscle toward the humerus. The cuff of triceps is left attached to the lateral intermuscular septum. Then the same is done from the anterior skin incision till a cuff of the brachialis muscle is left attached to the septum (see **Fig. 2.1**). The vascular pedicle may be traced, as already described, below the attachment of the deltoid muscle. The distal lateral part of the humeral shaft, whose attachment to the intermuscular septum is carefully preserved, is cut with an oscillating saw. Now the pedicle vessels (and nerve) are ligated and the flap is raised.

Primary wound closure may be attempted by mobilizing the borders. Skin grafting is required after harvesting large flaps. On grafting skin across the elbow joint, as in a lateral arm flap that extends into the proximal forearm, the elbow is immobilized in a semiflexed position for 2 weeks.

Pitfalls

Care is taken to isolate the radial nerve from the vascular pedicle and preserve it. It may look surprisingly easy to divide the septal connection of the bone segment in raising a composite flap; thus it is a good idea not to use a chisel to denude the bone, but to incise the periosteum at the site of the planned osteotomies. Large skin grafts extending across the elbow may be annoying: in the young due to the cosmetic appearance, and in the elderly due to possible postimmobilization stiffness of the elbow.

References

1 *Song R, Song Y, Yu Y, Song Y.* The upper arm free flap. Clin Plast Surg 1982;9:27–35

2 *Arnez ZM, Kersnic M, Smith RW, Godina M.* Free lateral arm osteocutaneous neurosensory flap for thumb reconstruction. J Hand Surg [Br] 1991;16:395–399

3 *Katsaros J, Schusterman M, Beppu M, Banis JC Jr, Acland RD.* The lateral upper arm flap: anatomy and clinical applications. Ann Plast Surg 1984;12:489–500

4 *Tan BK, Lim BH.* The lateral forearm flap as a modification of the lateral arm flap: vascular anatomy and clinical implications. Plast Reconstr Surg 2000;105:2400–2404

Chapter 3
The Radial Forearm Flap

The description of the free forearm flap based on the radial vessels in 1981 by Yang Guo-Fan and colleagues in the Chinese language,[1] some 3 years after its development, created a revolution in the use of free flaps. Until this time the use of free flaps was limited to a few "fathers" of the technique. Perhaps owing to the simple fact that the radial artery is known and palpated daily by all medical practitioners, the harvesting of this flap was made to appear uncomplicated. Thus the free flap transfer technique started to become popular not only among plastic surgeons, but also among other related specialties. Even today, the fasciocutaneous radial forearm flap serves as a workhorse in many hospitals, irrespective of the presence of a plastic surgeon in the team. The aphorism, "if all else fails, this is what you have to know," applies to the technique of harvesting the Chinese flap.

Preparation

A positive Allen test is a prerequisite for raising this flap: both the radial and the ulnar arteries are palpated at the wrist. Then both the arteries are occluded by applying pressure until one notices the hand turning pale from lack of circulation. Now the ulnar artery is opened, still holding the radial artery occluded. Brisk recirculation of the hand denotes the capability of perfusion via the ulnar artery alone, thus confirming the feasibility of harvesting the radial forearm flap. The patient is positioned supine, with the donor upper extremity spread on a hand table.

The forearm is kept in a supinated position. A nonexsanguinating tourniquet applied at the arm level is optional.

Neurovascular Anatomy

The radial artery is situated subcutaneously along most of its course through the anterolateral aspect of the forearm (**Fig. 3.1**). It is encompassed in the lateral intermuscular septum (deep fascia) that separates the flexor and extensor compartments of the forearm, the septum being attached to the periosteum of the radius distal to the insertion of the pronator teres tendon. The skin overlying the anterior aspect of the forearm is nourished by 7 to 14 perforating cutaneous arteries arising from the radial artery. Furthermore the branches of the radial artery supply the flexor and extensor muscles located in the vicinity, as well as the radial shaft. Although the dynamic perfusion territory of the radial flap is limited to the forearm skin, the potential perfusion territory is as large as three-quarters of the circumference of the forearm. Thus, if required, that much skin can be raised as a fasciocutaneous flap. The radial artery flap offers the possibility of harvesting it as a composite flap, with a segment of the distal radius and palmaris longus muscle.

This artery is provided with a pair of commitant veins, so that a distally based flap without additional subcutaneous venous anastomoses is possible.[2] The sensory innervation of the volar forearm skin overlying the radial artery is through the medial cutaneous nerve of the forearm. The lateral aspect is supplied by the lateral cutaneous nerve of the forearm, which is the sensory branch of the musculocutaneous nerve. One or both of these nerves may be raised with the flap to provide sensation in the recipient area.

Fig. 3.1 Vascular anatomy of the volar aspect of the forearm and hand.

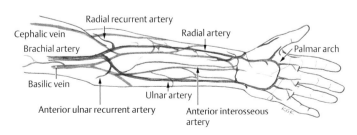

Radial recurrent artery
Cephalic vein
Brachial artery
Radial artery
Palmar arch
Basilic vein
Ulnar artery
Anterior ulnar recurrent artery
Anterior interosseous artery

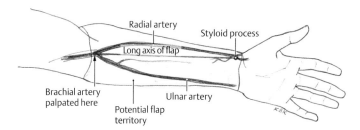

Fig. 3.2   Planning landmarks of the radial forearm flap.

Incisions and Dissection

With the forearm supinated, a straight line joining the middle of the cubital fossa (where the brachial artery is palpated) and the styloid process of radius is drawn (**Fig. 3.2**). This line denotes the course of the radial artery. The flap is centered along this axis. The ulnar border of the flap is incised until the deep fascia, preserving the sensory nerves and subcutaneous veins as required (**Fig. 3.3**). Dissection is then performed in the subfascial plane until the identification of the lateral intermuscular septum, where the radial vessels are encompassed. Now the vessels are dissected free from their perios-

teal attachments. The radial border of the flap is incised and the pedicle vessels approached, retracting the brachioradialis muscle. Here one encounters the radial nerve, which should be isolated and preserved. Skin incisions are made proximal and distal to the flap borders as required, to lengthen the vascular pedicle (**Fig. 3.4**). The radial artery may be ligated at its origin from the brachial, where its diameter amounts to around 3 mm.

If the harvesting of a composite flap is intended, then the radial vessels are not dissected free of their attachments to the radial periosteum. Instead, these are preserved, along with a cuff of surrounding muscles. A longitudinal os-

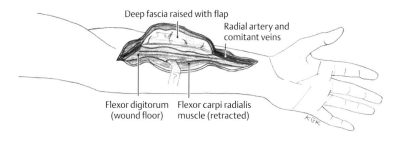

Fig. 3.3   Dissection of the radial forearm flap.

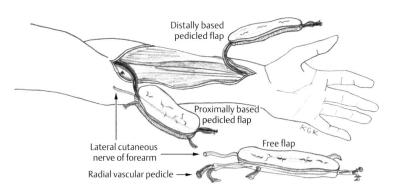

Fig. 3.4   Raising the radial forearm flap and its variations.

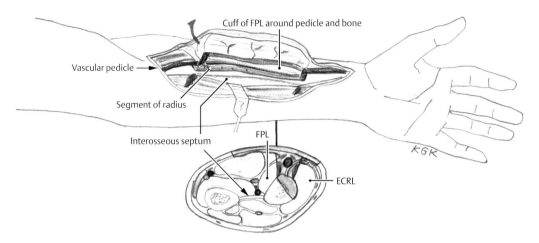

Fig. 3.5 Anatomical basis and raising of the osteocutaneous flap based on the radial artery. ECRL, extensor carpi radialis longus; FPL, flexor pollicis longus; U, ulna; R, radius.

teotomy of the distal segment of the radius is performed using an oscillating saw and this segment is raised as a component of the composite flap (**Fig. 3.5**). Direct closure may be attempted after raising small flaps; large flaps, however, require skin grafting.

There are two popular modifications in raising the radial forearm flap: namely, the suprafascial dissection technique[3] and the radial perforator flap.[4,5] While the suprafacial dissection technique serves to minimize donor tissue trauma, the distally based perforator flap aims at completely preserving the radial artery.

With the suprafascial dissection technique the skin incisions are performed on the ulnar side and the flap is raised in the suprafascial plane to ~1 cm distance from the lateral intermuscular septum, where the deep fascia is incised and included in the flap. Other aspects of dissection are the same as the technique described earlier.

The perforator flap is based on two or three major perforators arising from the radial artery ~2–4 cm above the styloid process. The skin incision is begun from the proximal margin of the flap and continues straight down to the deep

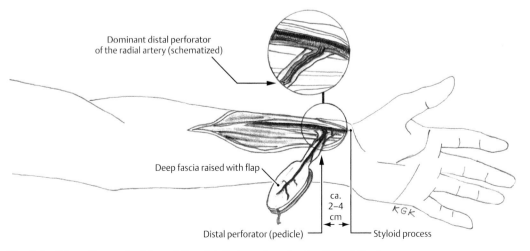

Fig. 3.6 Dissection and raising of the distally based perforator flap of the forearm.

fascia. The cephalic vein is ligated and divided at the proximal end. Then, the skin flap is elevated with deep fascia, along with the cephalic vein, leaving the radial artery intact (**Fig. 3.6**). The flap is dissected with a subcutaneous pedicle, 4 cm in width, which rises through the intertendinous septum between the brachioradialis and flexor carpi radialis tendon, from an S-shaped incision through the anterolateral aspect of the forearm. The proximal end of the subcutaneous pedicle is then transected, the septum near the radial vessels is dissected, and the perforators are carefully preserved. The proximal base of the pedicle is preserved as widely as possible, so there is no need for skeletonization of the perforators around the pivot point from the radial artery. The flap may be rotated now as a distally based island flap[5]; or, the pedicle is traced to its origin from the radial artery, which is divided and the flap raised as a free flap.[4]

> ### Pitfalls
>
> With a positive Allen test, there are no known major pitfalls in raising the radial forearm flap. Rarely, intraoperative occlusion of the radial artery might surprisingly show reduced hand perfusion. In this case, reconstruction of the radial artery using a reversed saphenous vein graft will be required. Skin grafts to the forearm after raising the flap may be cosmetically annoying. The sacrifice of the cutaneous nerves in raising sensate flaps is a disability that patients tolerate very well.

References

1 Yang GF, Chen PJ, Gao YZ, et al. Forearm free skin flap transplantation: a report of 56 cases. 1981. Br J Plast Surg 1997;50:162–165

2 Biemer E, Stock W. Total thumb reconstruction: a one-stage reconstruction using an osteo-cutaneous forearm flap. Br J Plast Surg 1983;36:52–55

3 Chang SC, Miller G, Halbert CF, Yang KH, Chao WC, Wei FC. Limiting donor site morbidity by suprafascial dissection of the radial forearm flap. Microsurgery 1996;17:136–140

4 Bauer TR, Schoeller T, Wechselberger G, Papp C. The radial artery perforator free flap. Plast Reconstr Surg 1999;104:885

5 Jeng SF, Wie FC. The distally based forearm island flap in hand reconstruction. Plast Reconstr Surg 1998;102:400–406

Chapter 4
The Ulnar Artery Free Flap

As an alternative to the radial forearm flap, the ulnar artery flap offers a thin and pliable cutaneous component as well as fascia in vascularized reconstructions of small defects. The free ulnar artery forearm flap was first described by Lovie et al. in 1984.[1] Since then it has continued to be a reliable, versatile, and convenient fasciocutaneous flap.[2,3] Flaps based on the medial aspect of the forearm are thin and hairless, thus making their application in intraoral or hand reconstructions attractive. Additionally the donor site of the ulnar artery flap is less obvious than its radial counterpart. In patients for whom only a small free flap with a short pedicle is necessary, the free ulnar artery forearm flap is technically straightforward and is quickly accomplished.

A flap based on the dorsal branch of the ulnar artery from the distal aspect of the forearm is described here.

Preparation

The ulnar artery is considered the lesser of the two major forearm arteries. However, as in preparing for the radial artery forearm flap, a positive Allen test is a required for raising the ulnar artery flap: both the radial and the ulnar arteries are palpated at the wrist. Both the arteries are then occluded by applying pressure until the hand turns noticeably pale from lack of circulation. Now the radial artery is opened, still holding the ulnar artery occluded. Brisk recirculation of the hand denotes the capability of perfusion via the radial artery alone, which is usually the case, and confirms the feasibility of harvesting the ulnar artery forearm flap. The patient is positioned supine, with the donor upper extremity spread on a hand table. The forearm is kept free to pronate or supinate as required during the course of raising the flap. A nonexsanguinating tourniquet applied at arm level is optional.

Neurovascular Anatomy

The dorsal branch of the ulnar artery and the dorsal branch of the ulnar nerve are constant structures. The dorsal branch of the ulnar artery originates ~4 cm (ranging between 2 and 7 cm) proximal to the pisiform bone. It can either emerge (most frequently) distally to the proximal limit of the pronator quadratus muscle, or proximally (**Fig. 4.1**). Rarely this vessel is a branch of the anterior interosseous artery. Anastomoses between the interosseous artery and the dorsal branch of the ulnar artery are found consistently along the insertion of the pronator quadratus muscle in the ulna. From this vascular arcade, several periosteal microvascular ramifications can be identified, thus providing the possibility of raising a portion of the ulnar bone as an osteocutaneous flap. More

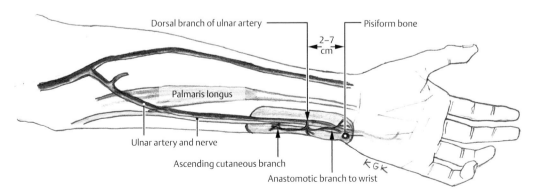

Fig. 4.1 Anatomical basis and planning markings of the forearm flap based on the dorsal branch of the ulnar artery.

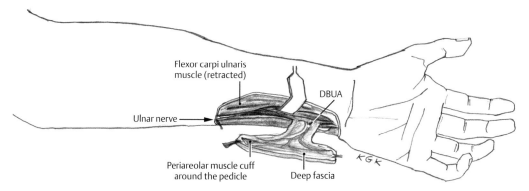

Flexor carpi ulnaris muscle (retracted)

DBUA

Ulnar nerve

Periareolar muscle cuff around the pedicle

Deep fascia

KGK

Fig. 4.2 Dissection and raising of the forearm flap based on the dorsal branch of the ulnar artery (DBUA).

distally along its course the dorsal branch of the ulnar artery divides into an ascending cutaneous branch, supplying the fasciocutaneous structures proximally, and a descending branch nourishing the skin of the dorsal ulnar aspect of the back of the hand, extending to the root of the little finger. A distally configured flap based on the distal microvascular anastomoses of this branch (with the dorsal intermetacarpal IV and palmar interdigital IV and V arteries) may be raised as a pedicled rotation flap,[3–5] whereas the proximally configured flap can be raised as a free flap.

The skin area achieves its sensory neural supply through the dorsal branch of the ulnar nerve that originates from the ulnar nerve ~6 cm (ranging between 5 and 16 cm) proximal to the pisiform bone. The course of this nerve is the same as that of the dorsal branch of the ulnar artery. Usually the nerve is located anterior to the artery. The nerve is vascularized by microvessels originating from the dorsal branch of the ulnar artery.

The diameter of the dorsal branch of the ulnar artery usually ranges from 0.8 and 1.5 mm at its origin and 0.5 mm at the level of the midcarpal articular line on the dorsal side of the wrist. The dorsal branch can also be traced to its origin from the ulnar artery, and a cuff of the ulnar artery can be harvested to ease microvascular manipulation. In this case the ends of the ulnar artery are mobilized in both directions and anastomosed to preserve circulation. The diameter of the dorsal branch of the ulnar nerve ranges between 1 and 3 mm at the point of its origin from the ulnar nerve.

Incisions and Dissection

With the forearm supinated, the pisiform eminence as well as the distal course of the ulnar bone are palpated and marked. The skin flap is centered on a point ~4–7 cm above the pisiform bone (**Fig. 4.1**). The anterior border of the skin is incised and the dissection is performed to the deep fascia covering the muscle structures. The fascia is incised and the fasciocutaneous segment is elevated to visualize the lateral border of the flexor carpi ulnaris muscle. Suitable perforators are identified within the septum passing between the flexor carpi ulnaris and flexor digitorum superficialis (**Fig. 4.2**). This perforator is traced to the ulnar artery located in the depth. Since the microvessels are quite delicate, it is a good idea to include a thin cuff of muscle tissue around the perforators. Then the ulnar artery is clamped, the tourniquet released, and the adequacy of hand perfusion is observed. Usually there is no change in hand perfusion on clamping the ulnar artery. The tourniquet is reinflated and the dorsal skin incisions are completed. A segment of the ulnar artery is raised with the pedicle and the ends of the ulnar artery are anastomosed to re-establish continuity. When a longer pedicle is required, the ulnar artery is mobilized proximally and raised with the flap. This would sacrifice the ulnar artery, usually without any consequence (**Figs. 4.3, 4.4**)

Depending on the amount of skin tissue raised, the donor wound is either closed primarily, after mobilizing the skin borders, or grafted. A length of superficial veins is raised

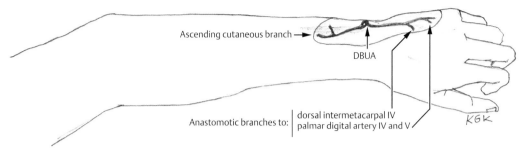

Fig. 4.3 Dorsal extension of the flap territory based on the dorsal branch of the ulnar artery (DBUA).

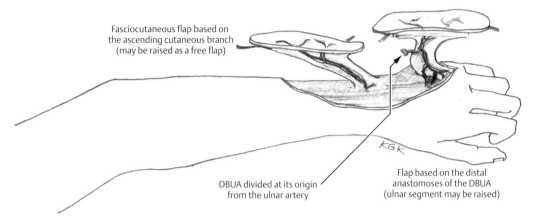

Fig. 4.4 Variations of the flap based on the dorsal branch of the ulnar artery (DBUA).

with the flap, to augment venous drainage at the recipient area as required.

When a more risky, distally pedicled flap based on the palmar arterial backflow of the ulnar artery is planned, then the distal cutaneous ramus of the vascular pedicle is traced and preserved; the proximal rami as well as the origin of the distal branch of the ulnar artery from the ulnar artery are divided between ligating clips (**Fig. 4.3**). The incisions of the skin flap are now completed and the flap may be rotated for reconstruction of fingers or the hand. Preserving a bridge of skin distally might reduce risks of lowered perfusion or venous stasis in the distally based flap.

Pitfalls

The distally pedicled flap based on the palmar arterial arch has risks of reduced perfusion or venous stasis, if the skin flap is circumferentially incised. Thus it might appear sensible to leave a bridge of skin intact at the base of the raised flap and correct the resulting "dog-ear" at a later stage.

References

1 *Lovie MJ, Duncan GM, Glasson DW.* The ulnar artery forearm free flap. Br J Plast Surg 1984;37:486–492

2 *Koshima I, Iino T, Fukuda H, Soeda S.* The free ulnar forearm flap. Ann Plast Surg 1987; 18:24–29

3 *Grobbelaar AO, Harrison DH.* The distally based ulnar artery island flap in hand reconstruction. J Hand Surg [Br] 1997;22:204–211

4 *Li ZT, Liu K, Cao Y.* The reverse flow ulnar artery island flap: 42 clinical cases. Br J Plast Surg 1989;42:256–259

5 *Yii NW, Niranjan NS.* Fascial flaps based on perforators for reconstruction of defects in the distal forearm. Br J Plast Surg 1999; 52:534–540

Chapter 5
The Posterior Interosseous Flap

A fasciocutaneous flap based on the posterior interosseous artery was first described by A.C. Masquelet. Penteado et al.[1] studied the anatomical basis of the posterior interosseous flap, confirmed the presence of this artery in 100 percent of cases, and verified the constancy of the pattern of integumentary perforators arising from this flap. Since then several modifications have been proposed.[2] The posterior interosseous flap may be transferred as a distally based pedicled island flap, in which case the blood supply follows the pathway of the recurrently perfused posterior interosseous artery through its distal anastomosis with the anterior interosseous artery,[3] or as a proximally based free flap. As for the tissue types, it is possible to raise the radial side of the midportion of the ulnar bone along with the fasciocutaneous flap— a valuable method for the reconstruction of a metacarpal bone associated with soft tissue loss.[2-5] The anatomical localization and the quality and types of tissue available for transfer make this flap a good option for hand resurfacing and reconstruction. Since both the major arteries of the forearm are left intact when raising the posterior interosseous flap, this flap may be considered as a minimally invasive alternative to the distally based radial forearm flap, which is also frequently used in hand reconstruction.

Preparation

The patient is positioned supine, with the upper extremity spread on a hand table. The forearm is kept in a fully pronated position. A nonexsanguinating tourniquet is applied at arm level both to facilitate bloodless dissection and eventually to raise subcutaneous veins draining the flap as required.

Neurovascular Anatomy

The skin overlying the posterior aspect of the forearm is nourished by 7 to 14 perforating cutaneous arteries arising from the posterior interosseous artery, which is a constant finding in all humans. This artery and its commitant veins—and additionally, in raising large flaps, the subcutaneous veins—serve as the basis of the fasciocutaneous flap described here. The sensation of this skin area is achieved through the posterior cutaneous nerve of the forearm, which is a sensory division of the radial nerve.

The posterior interosseous artery is one of the two branches of the common interosseous artery, which arises from the ulnar artery immediately below the radial tuberosity and passes backward toward the upper border of the interosseous membrane (**Figs. 5.1, 5.2**). In most cases a nerve fascicle runs across the posterior interosseous artery and subsequently into the extensor carpi ulnaris muscle. Behind the interosseous membrane the posterior interosseous artery appears between the contiguous borders of the supinator and the abductor pollicis longus; it runs down the back of the forearm between the superficial and deep layers of mus-

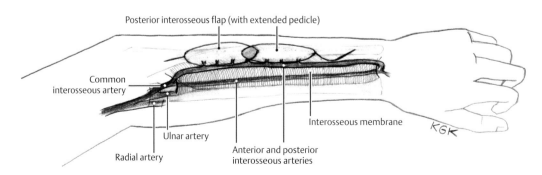

Posterior interosseous flap (with extended pedicle)

Common interosseous artery

Ulnar artery

Radial artery

Anterior and posterior interosseous arteries

Interosseous membrane

KGK

Fig. 5.1   Anatomical basis and skin markings of the posterior interosseous flap.

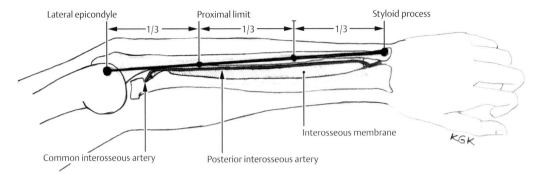

Lateral epicondyle   Proximal limit   Styloid process

|← 1/3 →|← 1/3 →|← 1/3 →|

Interosseous membrane

KGK

Common interosseous artery   Posterior interosseous artery

Fig. 5.2 Planning the posterior interosseous flap.

cles, distributing branches to these muscle layers as well as giving off cutaneous perforators through the septum between the extensor carpi ulnaris and the extensor digiti minimi muscles. It is accompanied by the posterior interosseous nerve, the motor deep branch of the radial nerve, along its course over the abductor pollicis longus and the extensor pollicis brevis. At the lower part of the forearm it runs forward toward the lower border of the interosseous membrane to anastomose with the termination of the anterior interosseous artery, and with the dorsal carpal arterial network.

Incisions and Dissection

With the forearm in full pronation, a straight line joining the lateral humeral epicondyle and the ulnar head is drawn. This line denotes the course of the posterior interosseous artery. The artery emerges at the posterior compartment of the forearm at the point bordering the proximal and middle thirds of this line. Proximal dissection should not exceed this point (**Fig. 5.2**). The important middle septocutaneous perforator of the posterior interosseous artery is situated at the midpoint of this line, thus the skin island is marked around this point in an oval pattern. The maximal size of the skin flap is 12 × 8 cm

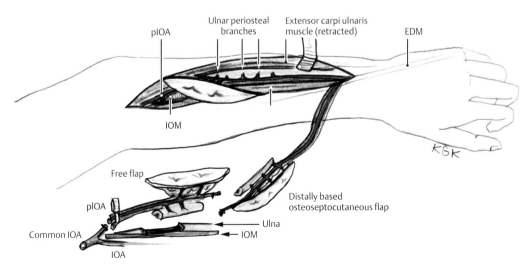

Ulnar periosteal   Extensor carpi ulnaris
plOA   branches   muscle (retracted)   EDM

IOM

Free flap

plOA   Distally based
osteoseptocutaneous flap

Ulna

Common IOA   IOM

IOA

Fig. 5.3 Dissection and raising of the posterior interosseous flap and some of its variations. EDM, extensor digiti minimi; IOA, interosseous artery; pIOA, posterior interosseous artery; aIOA, anterior interosseous artery; IOM, interosseous membrane.

along the axial line. The optimal flap configuration is 6 × 5 cm.

First, the distal incision is made and the extensor carpi ulnaris and extensor digiti minimi muscles/tendons are identified. The deep fascia is incised in such a way (including the paratendons of the above mentioned tendons) as to include the septum between these muscles. Here the posterior interosseous artery is identified and followed proximally until the distal border of the supinator muscle. Now the ulnar border of the skin flap is incised until the deep fascia and the dissection is performed in the subfascial plane toward the posterior interosseous artery, retracting the flexor carpi ulnaris muscle (**Fig. 5.3**). The radial border of the skin island is then incised and the posterior interosseous artery is identified from this approach retracting the extensor pollicis longus muscle. The posterior interosseous artery is divided as near to the supinator muscle as possible. Care is taken to identify the posterior interosseous nerve here and preserve it. The anterior connections of the artery are divided, which completes the dissection of the fasciocutaneous flap.

If it is intended to raise an osteofasciocutaneous flap, then the last step described above is performed differently. Instead of retracting the extensor pollicis longus muscle through the radial approach to the posterior interosseous artery, the dissection is extended deeper through a cuff of this muscle toward the interosseous membrane, which is divided along the intended length of bone harvest. From the side of the ulnar approach the broad posterior surface of the ulna is then exposed by dissecting through the muscle. The radial border of the ulna is cut using a power saw. Thus the fasciocutaneous flap, and posterior interosseous artery with a muscle cuff around it, along with a segment of the ulna, are raised as a composite flap (**Fig. 5.3**).

In raising a sensate flap, the posterior cutaneous nerve of the forearm that is encountered superficially as one makes the proximal skin incisions is followed further proximally, divided, marked and raised with the flap. Large flaps may require skin grafting. Otherwise primary closure is possible.

Pitfalls

It is important to identify and preserve the posterior interosseous nerve at the distal border of the supinator muscle. It is astonishingly easy to sever the arterial connection to the bone in raising the osteofasciocutaneous flap. Thus care and time should be taken to preserve these connections of the vascular pedicle. It is not a good idea to plan large flaps based on the posterior interosseous artery, for fear of partial necrosis. An augmenting venous anastomosis may be required in such conditions.

References

1 *Penteado CV, Masquelet AC, Chevrel JP.* The anatomic basis of the fascio-cutaneous flap of the posterior interosseous artery. Surg Radiol Anat 1986;8:209–215
2 *Cavadas PC.* Posterior interosseous free flap with extended pedicle for hand reconstruction. Plast Reconstr Surg 2001;108:897–901
3 *Angrigiani C, Grilli D, Dominikow D, Zancolli EA.* Posterior interosseous reverse forearm flap: experience with 80 consecutive cases. Plast Reconstr Surg 1993;92:285–293
4 *Costa H, Smith R, McGrouther DA.* Thumb reconstruction by the posterior interosseous osteocutaneous flap. Br J Plast Surg 1988; 41:228–233
5 *Akin S, Ozgenel Y, Ozcan M.* Osteocutaneous posterior interosseous flap for reconstruction of the metacarpal bone and soft-tissue defects in the hand. Plast Reconstr Surg 2002;109:982–987

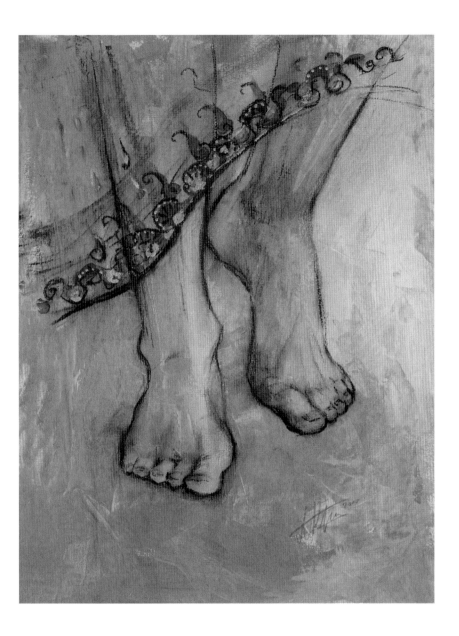

Part 2
Flaps of the Lower Extremity

Part 2
Flaps of the Lower Extremity

The lower extremity offers a variety of soft-tissue and bone flaps to meet challenging reconstructive problems. Many flaps may be raised for free microvascular transfer (gracilis, fibula, dorsal foot, free toe), while some others find adequate application as local pedicled rotation flaps (gastrocnemius, saphenous, superficial sural artery, medial plantar, etc.).

Several of these flaps have specific properties peculiar to them alone; for instance, the possibility of motor innervation in the gracilis, the availability of an articular surface of the metatarsal bone, etc. These properties are favorably harnessed to meet specific reconstructive requirements.

The outstanding reconstructive microsurgeon considers the specific and nonspecific demands of the recipient defect and chooses an optimal flap to attain adequate coverage, restore function, and render the site an aesthetic appearance that is as pleasing as possible. Lower extremity flaps are very advantageous in several respects: the harvest of most of the flaps from the lower extremity does not greatly disadvantage the day-to-day life of the patient. Moreover, the donor site is clothed most of the time, thus saving social embarrassment.

In this section I have described seven different flaps and their variations. Naturally, the lower extremity has much more to offer than these seven, but the presentation is limited to flaps that are reliable. The mastery of these flaps through repeated anatomical study in cadavers, active participation in the performance in patients, and, importantly, review of the up-to-date literature before attending to each case, will offer assuredness to the trainee that will open new options in every subsequent case she or he attends. After all, reconstructive surgery demands a high level of innovative thinking and a sound working knowledge of the relevant normal anatomy for carrying out such "unusual" procedures in a safe manner.

Chapter 6
The Gracilis Muscle Flap

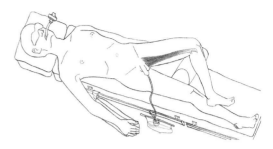

The gracilis muscle as a free vascularized flap was first described by Harii, Ohmori, and Torii in 1976.[1,2] According to the classification of Mathes and Nahai (see Chapter 21), the gracilis muscle receives a type 2 vascular supply (one dominant pedicle and other minor pedicles). Based on its innervation, the muscle could be divided into two surgical units, an anterior and a posterior one.[3] It is important to differentiate this division, especially in transferring a split gracilis free innervated flap for facial reanimation.

The gracilis muscle has a constant vascular supply and innervation, and leaves behind a relatively negligible functional loss at the donor site. These properties make it a favorite flap in hand and facial reanimation. The muscle is less reliable as a musculocutaneous flap, since the vascular supply of the skin overlying the gracilis muscle is quite variable. A skin paddle designed longitudinally on the most proximal part of the musculocutaneous flap, and of dimensions less than 6 × 7 cm should, as a rule, survive.

Preparation

The patient is positioned supine, with the donor lower extremity gently flexed at the knee and externally rotated and flexed at the hip

Fig. 6.1 Patient positioning for the harvest of the gracilis flap.

joint, making the approach to the muscle straightforward (**Fig. 6.1**). No myorelaxants are administered until the flap harvest is completed, since at the end of the flap harvest the innervating nerve (anterior branch of the obturator nerve) will be stimulated to identify the fascicles of the nerve that are to be sutured to the motor nerve at the recipient site. Accumulation of myorelaxants in the harvested muscle tissue would mask a motor response upon direct nerve stimulation.

Neurovascular Anatomy

The gracilis muscle originates from a soft-tissue aponeurosis beneath and behind the palpable pubic symphysis; it courses along the inner thigh and inserts into the medial part of the tibial metaphysis (**Fig. 6.2**). Here, a thin tendinous slip may separate and turn dorsally to insert into the crural deep fascia. The muscle is not directly palpable, especially in muscular patients, in whom the mass of the adductors may overlap

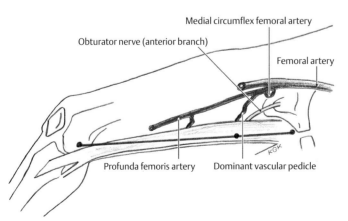

Medial circumflex femoral artery
Obturator nerve (anterior branch)
Femoral artery
Profunda femoris artery   Dominant vascular pedicle

Fig. 6.2 Anatomical basis of the gracilis flap.

Fig. 6.3 Planning markings of the gracilis flap.

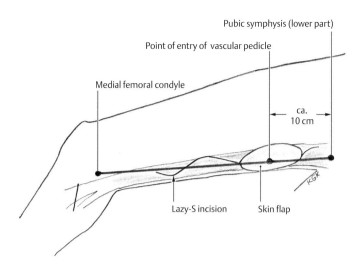

Pubic symphysis (lower part)

Point of entry of vascular pedicle

Medial femoral condyle

ca. 10 cm

Lazy-S incision   Skin flap

the gracilis. The approximate course of the muscle is traced by drawing a straight line connecting the pubic symphysis and the medial femoral condyle. The muscle is nourished by three or four, more or less equivalent vascular pedicles that arise from the deep femoral vessels. The most proximal pedicle is the major vascular nourisher. This artery arises either from the medial circumflex femoral artery or, a little distally, directly from the profunda femoris artery. Then it travels along the space between the adductor longus (anterior to the pedicle) and adductor magnus (lies posteriorly), and enters the gracilis muscle belly at a point ~6–12 cm below the muscle origin (**Fig. 6.3**). The skin overlying the gracilis muscle at this point is supplied by perforating vessels arising from the major vascular pedicle. More distally the skin is nourished through vessels originating from the anterior thigh region. The nerve that renders motor innervation to the muscle is the anterior branch of the obturator nerve. The nerve enters the muscle belly in the same coronal plane as the vessels, but ~1 cm more proximally. This nerve, as a rule, is composed of four fascicles, one of them being larger than the others. The larger fascicle innervates the anterior portion of the gracilis muscle. In transferring a split gracilis free flap, it is important to recognize this by direct nerve stimulation, and to suture the corresponding fascicles to the motor nerve at the recipient site.

Incisions and Dissection

If there is need to transfer the muscle as a musculocutaneous flap, the skin paddle is marked as follows: a straight line is drawn from the lower aspect of the pubic symphysis to the medial femoral condyle (**Fig. 6.3**). Approximately 10 cm distal to the starting point of the line denotes the point of entry of the vascular pedicle into the muscle belly, and consecutively also of the skin perforator, which can be examined using a hand-held Doppler. The skin flap has a maximum dimension of 6 × 7 cm designed longitudinally along the proximal portion of the muscle flap. A longer skin paddle may develop partial distal necrosis after transfer. This is true, even if a secondary vascular pedicle is anastomosed at the recipient site.

The anterior skin incisions are made first, extending the cut in the form of a lazy-S, both proximally and distally as needed. The deep fascia is sharply cut and the anterior border of the gracilis muscle identified. When the anterior border of the gracilis muscle has been exposed through blunt dissection, the neurovascular pedicle may be identified by gently retracting the muscle medially and dorsally. The vascular pedicle is followed by blunt separation of the septal plane between the adductor longus and adductor magnus muscles to its origin. From the surgeon's view, one sees the neurovascular pedicle lying on the adductor magnus, as the assistant retracts the adductor longus above

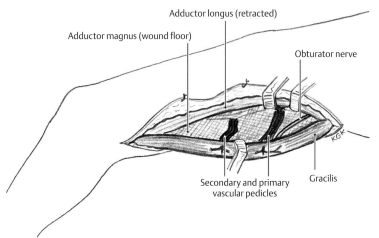

Fig. 6.4 Dissection of the gracilis flap.

Adductor longus (retracted)

Adductor magnus (wound floor)

Obturator nerve

Secondary and primary vascular pedicles

Gracilis

(**Fig. 6.4**). Now the anterior border of the muscle is followed distally until the end of the incision. One may encounter the secondary, tertiary, and even the quaternary pedicles of the muscle along the way. If the caliber of the vessels matches the major proximal pedicle, then the pedicle is also raised along the flap. But if the pedicle contains significantly smaller vessels, then it is divided sharply between ligatures. Before releasing the tendon, the leg is positioned so that the gracilis muscle is stretched to its maximum, and marking sutures, spaced 5 cm apart, are placed on the muscle border (**Fig. 6.5**). These sutures serve as a guideline as to the amount of linear tension with which the muscle should be fixed in the recipient site. When a split muscle flap is to be transplanted, then the nerve fascicles are stimulated, and the motor fascicle corresponding to the muscle division to be transferred is marked with an 8/0 suture. The tendon of the muscle is released through an ancillary incision placed over the medial side of the tibial head. Now the posterior skin incision for raising the musculocutaneous flap is completed. The muscle is then released from its posterior septal and fascial attachments. The proximal origin of the muscle is sharply transected. At this point, the only remaining connections of the flap to the body are through the neurovascular pedicle. By retract-

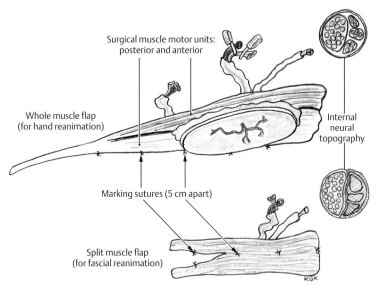

Fig. 6.5 The harvested gracilis flap and its variations.

Surgical muscle motor units: posterior and anterior

Whole muscle flap (for hand reanimation)

Internal neural topography

Marking sutures (5 cm apart)

Split muscle flap (for fascial reanimation)

ing the adductor longus, the pedicle is followed as proximally as possible. The artery and the veins are ligated separately before dividing the pedicle. The nerve is traced to its exit from the obturator foramen, ligated proximally, and divided. Donor site closure is made on primary intention by mobilizing the skin borders, after placing a suction drain in the dead space created by the harvested muscle.

The major vascular pedicle is usually 5–6 cm long. The artery and the vein have diameters of ~1.5–2 mm and 2–3 mm, respectively. As a rule the neural pedicle is comparable in length to the vascular one.

The results of innervated and vascularized gracilis muscle transfer are found to be favorable, especially when the nerve suture is performed as near to the muscle flap as possible.

Pitfalls

In a musculocutaneous flap, it is important to design the skin paddle on the proximal part of the gracilis muscle. There are reports on the intraoperative usage of fluorescine dye to demarcate the perfused skin island under a blue light filter. The intravenous administration of this substance is not permitted in certain countries (for instance, Germany). An excessively large skin flap may fail, while the muscle remains adequately perfused.

In transplanting a split muscle, it is necessary to identify the nerve fascicle that innervates the muscle division to be transferred and mark it.

The tension with which the muscle is fixed in the recipient site should be determined before releasing the flap in the donor site, and marked with sutures placed equidistant from each other. Inadequate tension of the muscle at the recipient site may mandate a separate lifting operation at a later stage.

References

1 *Harii K, Ohmori K, Torii S.* Free gracilis muscle transplantation, with microneurovascular anastomoses for the treatment of facial paralysis. A preliminary report. Plast Reconstr Surg 1976;57:133–143

2 *Harii K, Ohmori K, Sekiguchi J.* The free musculocutaneous flap. Plast Reconstr Surg 1976;57:294–303

3 Manktelow RT. Microneurovascular free muscle transfer. In: Omer GE Jr, Spinner M, Van Beek AL, eds. *Management of Peripheral Nerve Problems*. Philadelphia, Pa: WB Saunders; 1998:731–743.

Chapter 7
The Tensor Fasciae Latae Muscle Flap

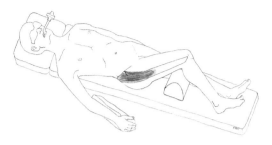

Fig. 7.1   Patient positioning for the harvest of the tensor fasciae latae flap.

The tensor fasciae latae muscle arises from the anterior part of the outer lip of the iliac crest and is invested in a double fascial layer. These fascial layers blend at the junction between the upper and the middle thirds of the lateral aspect of the thigh and course down as the ilio-tibial tract to insert into the lateral femoral condyle. The muscle flexes and rotates the femur internally.

The muscle is provided with a constant blood supply through one reliable vascular pedicle arising from the lateral circumflex femoral artery and its accompanying vein. The motor innervation is through the descending branch of the superior gluteal nerve. The overlying skin has two sources of sensory innervation: (1) the cutaneous branch of the T12 segment (upper part), and (2) the lateral femoral cutaneous nerve (lower part).

The tensor fasciae latae was first described as a free musculocutaneous flap by Hill, Nahai, and Vasconez in 1978.[1,2] This musculocutaneous unit can be transferred with motor as well as sensory innervation; there are ample and different types of tissue that may be transferred based on the vascular pedicle of this muscle.[3–6] These properties make the tensor fasciae latae muscle a very reliable workhorse for dealing with various reconstructive challenges.[4,6]

Preparation

If not otherwise dictated by the site to be reconstructed, the patient is positioned supine with the hip and knee joints gently flexed. The thigh is rotated internally, so that its lateral aspect faces the surgeon (**Fig. 7.1**). The anterior superior iliac spine and the iliac crest are palpated and marked. The line joining the lateral most aspect of the iliac crest and the lateral femoral condyle marks the course of the iliotibial tract.

The position of the patient is determined by the area to be reconstructed. For instance, in using the tensor fasciae latae muscle as a pedicled rotation flap for the reconstruction of decubitus wounds, the patient may be positioned either on the side or in a prone posture.

Neurovascular Anatomy (Fig. 7.2)

The vascular pedicle that nourishes the tensor fasciae latae muscle arises either from the lateral circumflex femoral artery or, in some cases,

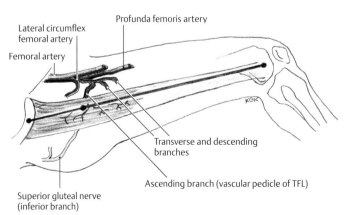

Fig. 7.2   Anatomical basis of the tensor faciae latae (TFL) flap.

Lateral circumflex femoral artery

Profunda femoris artery

Femoral artery

Transverse and descending branches

Ascending branch (vascular pedicle of TFL)

Superior gluteal nerve (inferior branch)

Fig. 7.3 Planning markings of the tensor faciae latae flap.

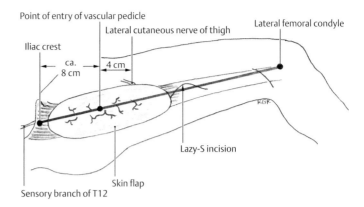

directly from the profunda femoris artery as an ascending branch. The pedicle enters the muscle belly ~6–8 cm distal to the muscle's origin from the iliac crest. The skin overlying the muscle is richly vascularized by about four or five perforator vessels arising from this vascular pedicle.

The motor innervation is executed from the dorsal aspect through the descending branch of the superior gluteal nerve. The sensory innervation of the overlying skin is accomplished by the cutaneous branch of T12 that enters the lateral thigh region after crossing the iliac crest, and by the lateral femoral cutaneous nerve that enters the anterior border of the lateral thigh skin ~10–12 cm distal to the origin of the tensor fasciae latae muscle.

The vascular pedicle as well as the motor and sensory nerves can be reliably dissected by orienting oneself on the landmarks as described later.

Incisions and Dissection

The iliac crest, the anterior iliac superior spine, as well as the lateral femoral condyle are palpated and marked. A straight line joining the lateral-most aspect of the iliac crest and the lateral femoral condyle mark the approximate course of the musculofascial tract (**Fig. 7.3**). Moreover, the muscle belly is palpated and marked. If needs be, practically the whole of the skin of the lateral thigh may be raised along with the underlying muscle and fascia based on the single vascular pedicle.

A skin island centered along the tensor fasciae latae muscle belly is described here. Two

points, 8 and 10 cm distal to the iliac crest and along the anterior muscle border, are marked. These represent the entry points of the vascular pedicle and the lateral femoral cutaneous nerve, respectively.

The anterior border of the skin flap is incised first, extending the incision in a lazy-S pattern proximally and distally as found necessary. Care is taken to preserve the lateral femoral cutaneous nerve that appears along the incision.

After the anterior border of the tensor fasciae latae muscle has been identified and dissected free, the muscle belly is retracted laterally and dorsally to reveal the entry point of the vascular pedicle (~6–8 cm distal to the muscle origin). These vessels travel in the septal space between the rectus femoris (anteriorly) and vastus lateralis muscle (posteriorly). Thus the rectus femoris is separated bluntly from the septal space and retracted anteromedially to visualize the course of the vascular pedicle (**Fig. 7.4**).

Now the posterior incisions of the skin island are completed, taking care to preserve the cutaneous nerve entering the skin island laterally along the iliac crest. The iliotibial tract is dissected and transected as distally as needed.

If the recipient site demands the transfer of a functional muscle, the dissection of the motor nerve is performed as follows: the posterior border of the muscle is freed sharply cut from the fascial attachments and the muscle is retracted anteromedially (**Fig. 7.5**). The gluteus medius muscle that inserts into the greater femoral trochanter is retracted posteriorly to reveal the motor nerve innervating the tensor

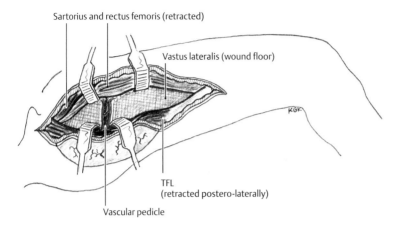

Sartorius and rectus femoris (retracted)

Vastus lateralis (wound floor)

KGK

TFL
(retracted postero-laterally)

Vascular pedicle

Fig. 7.4 Dissection of the tensor faciae latae (TFL) flap.

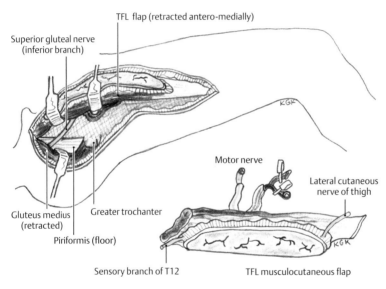

TFL flap (retracted antero-medially)

Superior gluteal nerve
(inferior branch)

KGK

Motor nerve

Lateral cutaneous
nerve of thigh

Gluteus medius   Greater trochanter
(retracted)

Piriformis (floor)

Sensory branch of T12

TFL musculocutaneous flap

KGK

Fig. 7.5 Harvesting the tensor faciae latae (TFL) flap.

fasciae latae muscle. This nerve courses between the piriformis (anteriorly) and the gluteus medius muscle (posteriorly). The nerve is now stimulated and transected after confirming the motor response from the muscle flap.

After the muscle or musculocutaneous flap has been cut, the vascular pedicle is followed to its origin, retracting the rectus femoris muscle anteromedially. The artery and veins are transected separately between ligating clips.

The vascular pedicle is ~6–8 cm in length; the vessel diameters are in the order of 2–2.5 mm (artery) and 3 mm (vein). Based on this single vascular pedicle it is possible and reliable to raise the whole of the iliotibial tract along with the overlying skin (~40 × 20 cm). The motor nerve is 1–1.5 mm in diameter and is relatively short in length (approx. 5 cm).

Disadvantages associated with raising a large tensor fasciae latae musculocutaneous flap include muscle herniation and a long scar. Skin grafting may be necessary, where a broad skin flap has been cut.

Pitfalls

Dissection of this usually reliable flap may be demanding when an innervated flap has been planned. Particular care is necessary during the posterior dissection, where the motor nerve runs. It is surprisingly easy to transect the innervating nerves, since these are relatively small in caliber and short in length. Some situations may demand a nerve graft between the donor nerve at the recipient site and the motor nerve of the flap, owing to the limited length of the motor nerve. In our experience results after transferring functional muscle flaps were better when no nerve grafts were used.

It is safe to transfer this flap without motor innervation. Recipient sites that definitively demand a motor innervated muscle may be better treated with the gracilis or latissimus dorsi muscle flaps instead of the tensor fasciae latae muscle.

References

1 *Hill HL, Nahai F, Vasconez LO.* The tensor fascia lata myocutaneous free flap. Plast Reconstr Surg 1978;61:517–522

2 *Nahai F, Silverton JS, Hill HL, Vasconez LO.* The tensor fascia lata musculocutaneous flap. Ann Plast Surg 1978;1:372–379

3 *Brenner P, Krebs C.* Brachial plexus innervated, functional tensor fasciae latae muscle transfer for controlling a Utah Arm after dislocation of the shoulder caused by an electrical burn. J Trauma 2001;50:562–567

4 *Deiler S, Pfadenhauer A, Widmann J, Stutzle H, Kanz KG, Stock W.* Tensor fasciae latae perforator flap for reconstruction of composite Achilles tendon defects with skin and vascularized fascia. Plast Reconstr Surg 2000; 106:342–349

5 *Ihara K, Doi K, Shigetomi M, Kawai S.* Tensor fasciae latae flap: alternative donor as a functioning muscle transplantation. Plast Reconstr Surg 1997;100:1812–1816

6 *Krishnan KG, Winkler PA, Müller A, Grevers G, Steiger HJ.* Closure of recurrent frontal skull base defects with vascularized flaps – a technical case report. Acta Neurochir (Wien) 2000;142:1353–1358

Chapter 8
The Gastrocnemius Muscle Flap

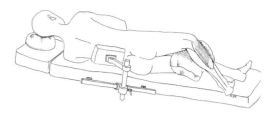

Fig. 8.1   Patient positioning for the harvest of the gastrocnemius flap.

The gastrocnemius muscle flap is probably the most preferred muscle or musculocutaneous flap for reconstruction of defects around the knee area. The transposition of lateral and medial heads of the gastrocnemius muscle were described by Barfod[1] and Ger,[2] respectively. Both heads of this muscle can be favorably used for various reconstructive procedures, since the sural vessels entering the respective muscle heads represent, more or less, a mirror image (Mathes and Nahai type 1 flap; see Chapter 21). The vascular anatomy is constant. Thus the flap may be raised, transposed, or transferred in a variety of ways: as a proximally or distally based flap,[3,4] as a free neurovascular flap,[5] or even as a rotation flap augmented by vascular anastomoses.[6] In bulky individuals one muscle head may be further split based on its intramuscular vascular ramification, and a part of the flap transposed.[7] Raising a proximally based gastrocnemius flap, which is considered the most reliable, is described here.

Preparation

The patient is placed in the lateral decubitus or in the prone position and the donor leg is draped in a mobile manner (**Fig. 8.1**). A tourniquet applied to the upper thigh may allow a bloodless dissection.

Neurovascular Anatomy

The gastrocnemius is a bicapitate muscle, the heads of which are connected to the femoral condyles by strong, flat tendons. Both heads run toward the midline of the calf to join each other, the medial head being a bit thicker and longer than the lateral one, thus providing a better radius of rotation. The muscle bellies unite at an angle in the midline of the muscle in a tendinous raphe, which expands into a broad aponeurosis on the anterior surface of the muscle. The aponeurosis unites with the tendon of the soleus, and forms with it the Achilles tendon. The cleft formed at the point of union of the two heads, the muscle bellies and the tendon are easily palpated and marked. The vascular supply is achieved through the lateral and medial sural arteries that arise from the popliteal artery and enter the muscle heads near to their origin (**Fig. 8.2**). Once having entered the muscle, the sural artery further divides and supplies several segments of the muscle belly, finally anastomosing with the sural artery of the other muscle belly. A working knowledge of this in-

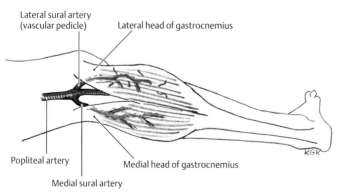

Lateral sural artery
(vascular pedicle)   Lateral head of gastrocnemius

Popliteal artery

Medial head of gastrocnemius

Medial sural artery

Fig. 8.2   Anatomical basis of the gastrocnemius flap.

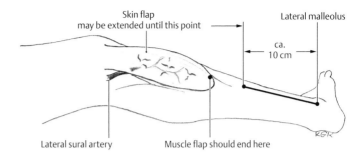

Fig. 8.3 Planning markings of the gastrocnemius flap.

tramuscular vascular tree makes it possible to split one belly of the gastrocnemius muscle and rotate it, or, alternatively, design a distally based flap for covering defects of the shin region. The nerve supply is through the motor fascicles leaving the tibial nerve, not unlike the sural arteries arising from the popliteal artery. The skin overlying the muscle is nourished by numerous perforator vessels.

Incisions and Dissection

The technique of raising a proximally based flap is described here. The courses of the muscle heads are easily palpated and marked. The muscle can be raised until the point where it turns tendinous. The overlying skin, however, may be cut as distal as 10 cm above the respective malleolus when a musculocutaneous flap is called for (**Fig. 8.3**). Skin flaps designed longer should theoretically survive, since the potential territories tend to expand after raising a flap. But this is not always safe in practice.

The midline incision is made first and the cleft formed by fusion of the gastrocnemius heads exposed, taking care to preserve the sural nerve during the subcutaneous dissection. By retracting the two heads gently apart, the vessels entering the muscle belly to be raised are visualized and separated using a vessel loop (this maneuver is actually not necessary if the radius of rotation does not exceed 100°). Now the muscle is sharply separated from the raphe and raised with the sheath in which the muscle is invested (**Fig. 8.4**). In using a musculocutaneous flap, a longer skin flap may be raised, the width not exceeding the muscle bulk (maximally 30 × 8 cm). The distal skin incision is made and dissection performed in a plane below the deep fascia in the proximal direction until the muscle belly is visualized. From then on, the skin is never separated from the muscle, and the dissection is performed bluntly in the submuscular (gastrocnemius) plane after dividing the muscle fibers from their distal connections. As long as the nourishing vessels and their entry into the muscle are kept under direct vision and their integrity respected, mobilization may be performed as proximally as possible. A radius of rotation of 100° should still not cause kinking of the vessels if the head of gastrocnemius is left attached to the femoral

Fig. 8.4 Dissection of the gastrocnemius flap.

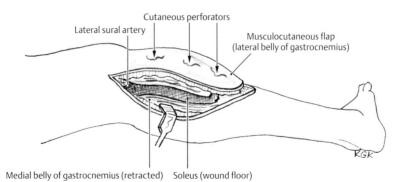

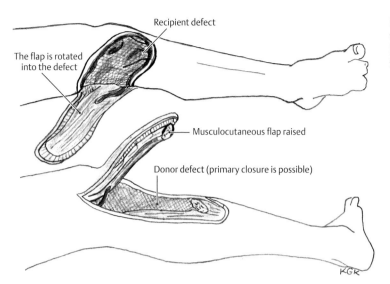

Recipient defect

The flap is rotated into the defect

Musculocutaneous flap raised

Donor defect (primary closure is possible)

Fig. 8.5 An example of wound closure with the harvested gastrocnemius flap.

condyle (**Fig. 8.5**). If more rotation is called for, it is wise to release the head of gastrocnemius, care being taken to preserve the vascular pedicle.

In raising the gastrocnemius as a free flap, the vessels are divided at their junction with the popliteal vessels. The motor nerve entering the gastrocnemius head can be found when dissecting the vascular structures. This nerve is traced to its origin from the tibial nerve and divided there. Fascicular neurolysis of the tibial nerve at this region might add an extra centimeter to the length of the nerve. The vessels are quite large (2.5–3 mm in diameter) and the pedicle is ~5 cm long (3–8 cm).

Pitfalls

The sural nerve surfaces to the subcutaneous plane approximately at the point of junction of the two gastrocnemius heads. Care should be taken to preserve this nerve during the initial skin incisions. Failure to do so will result in a respective sensory loss.

In heavily muscular individuals, the bulkiness of the muscle can be excessive, which both hinders muscle rotation and causes bulging. To overcome these drawbacks, advantage may be taken of the intramuscular arterial anatomy and the muscle may further be split longitudinally.[7] However, the arch of rotation remains limited with this modification.

In using a distally based flap, the raphe is kept intact as far as possible. Too much mobilization might divide the tiny, but important, anastomoses between the lateral and medial sural arterial systems.[3,8] If, after releasing the tourniquet, the distally based flap does not seem to bleed adequately, flap vascularity may be augmented by suturing the sural vessels raised with the flap to the vessels of the recipient area.[6]

References

1 *Barfod B, Pers M.* Gastrocnemius-plasty for primary closure of compound injuries of the knee. J Bone Joint Surg Br 1970;52: 124–127

2 *Ger R.* The technique of muscle transposition in the operative treatment of traumatic and ulcerative lesions of the leg. J Trauma 1971; 11:502–510

3 *Atchabahian A, Masquelet AC.* The distally based medial gastrocnemius flap: case report and anatomic study. Plast Reconstr Surg 1996;98:1253–1257

4 *Bashir AH.* Inferiorly-based gastrocnemius muscle flap in the treatment of war wounds of the middle and lower third of the leg. Br J Plast Surg 1983;36:307–309

5 *Liu XY, Ge BF, Win YM, Jing H.* Free medial gastrocnemius myocutaneous flap transfer with neurovascular anastomosis to treat Volk-

mann's contracture of the forearm. Br J Plast Surg 1992;45:6–8

6 Chen HC, Tang YB, Noordhoff MS. Distally based gastrocnemius myocutaneous flap augmented with an arterial anastomosis – a combination of myocutaneous flap and microsurgery. J Trauma 1988;28:110–114

7 Pedro C, Cavadas PC. The split medial gastrocnemius muscle flap. Plast Reconstr Surg 1998;102:1782–1783

8 Tsetsonis CH, Kaxira OS, Laoulakos DH, Spiliopoulou CA, Koutselinis AS. The inferiorly based gastrocnemius muscle flap: anatomic aspects. Plast Reconstr Surg 2000;106:1312–1315

Chapter 9
The Vascularized Fibula Flap

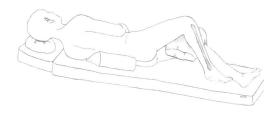

Fig. 9.1   Patient positioning for the harvest of the fibula flap.

Since its first description as a vascularized bone graft,[1,2] the fibula has continued to serve in meeting a variety of reconstructive challenges.[3-6] The fibula offers excellent tricortical bone tissue that has a reliable vascular pedicle and could also be raised as an osteoseptocutaneous flap for combined bone and integumentary reconstruction. Nourished by the peroneal vessels in an intramedullary as well as in a periosteal fashion, this flap is quite tolerant to osteotomies, still remaining nicely vascularized.[5,7,8] The long-term results of both the effect of vascularized transfer of the fibular shaft and the morbidity caused by its harvest are well studied, thus making this flap a safe option.[4,9]

There is a report on the transfer of fibula along with its epiphyseal plate for the reconstruction of the proximal humerus in a growing boy.[10] However, the author describes the use of a separate second pedicle to vascularize the fibular head and its growth plate. The results are impressive and there seems no additional morbidity associated with the harvest of the fibular head,[10] a sensitive topic for those who have not used this technique. But this method is yet to stand the test of time and experience.

In this chapter, we will discuss the anatomy and the vascularized harvest of the fibular shaft as an osteoseptocutaneous flap.

Preparation

The positioning of the patient may be varied to advantage with respect to the exposure of the site to be reconstructed. A semi-lateral decubitus position with the back supported by a wedge-shaped pillow and the donor leg gently flexed at the knee and rotated internally will make the approach straightforward (**Fig. 9.1**). However, the approach can be made equally comfortable in a supine or a prone patient, supporting the lower extremity respectively in an internally or externally rotated position. An ex-

sanguinating tourniquet is applied at the upper thigh and the extremity draped in a mobile manner, so as to vary the limb position intraoperatively as required.

Vascular Anatomy (Fig. 9.2)

The fibular shaft has a reliable vascular pedicle (peroneal vessels) with very little variation of its topographical anatomy. The peroneal artery arises from the posterior tibial artery behind the interosseous septum, ~2.5 cm below the lower border of the popliteus muscle; it passes obliquely toward the fibula, and then descends along the medial side of the bone, and is contained in a fibrous canal between the tibialis posterior and the flexor hallucis longus muscles. In the upper and middle parts of its course, the artery gives out tiny branches that circumvent the fibula, and run along the lateral crural intermuscular septum to supply the skin overlying the fibula. These vessels serve as the basis for an osteoseptocutaneous flap.

As a variation, the peroneal artery may arise 7 or 8 cm below the popliteus muscle, or from the posterior tibial artery high up, or rarely, even directly from the popliteal artery. It is extremely unlikely that the peroneal artery is entirely absent.

Approximately at the proximal part of the middle third of the fibula, a large, proper nutrient artery enters the medullary canal. The periosteum of the bone receives numerous vessels all along the course of the peroneal artery. Thus the vasculature is twofold: intramedullary and periosteal. One may take good advantage of this peculiarity and bench-modify the fibular shaft as required with multiple osteotomies, importantly preserving the periosteal connection be-

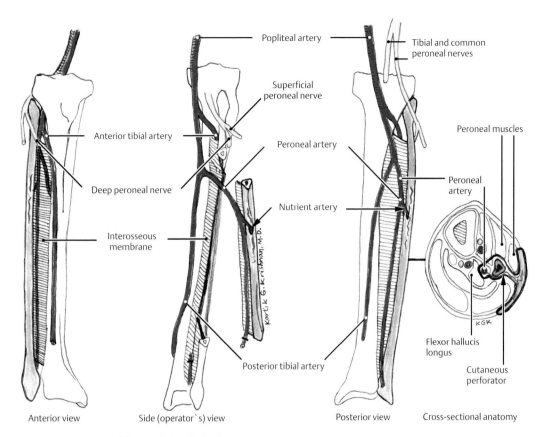

Fig. 9.2   Anatomical basis of the fibula flap.

tween the bone segments that assures adequate vascularity of the resulting flap.

Incisions and Dissection

The course of fibula is palpated along the lateral leg and marked. Then the length is divided into three equal parts. The fibular nutrient artery enters the medial aspect of the bone somewhere in the proximal part of the middle segment (**Fig. 9.3**). If the harvest of a skin paddle along the bone flap is called for, then the skin island is marked as an ellipse along the long axis of the fibula, so that it lies approximately over the proximal/middle third of the bone. The cutaneous perfusion will prove sufficient if the skin-flap dimensions do not exceed 8 cm in width, although larger flaps have been reported to survive.[6]

A posterior border of the skin flap is incised until the deep fascia, including the latter with the skin island, and the incision is extended both proximally and distally in a lazy-S pattern. Distal to the skin flap the skin borders are retracted and blunt dissection is performed till the bone. The bone is freed from all its attachments along its entire circumference at the point of osteotomy (this should be at least 6 cm proximal to the ankle joint). Failure to preserve enough bone length distally would lead to joint instability. A Gigli bone saw is passed around the fibula and the bone is divided. The peroneal vessels are readily visualized as the cut fibula is laterally distracted. The vessels are ligated and divided here. Then the dissection is proceeded in the proximal direction, incising the interosseous septum with scissors and keeping the vessels under direct vision (Fig. 9.4). The tibial

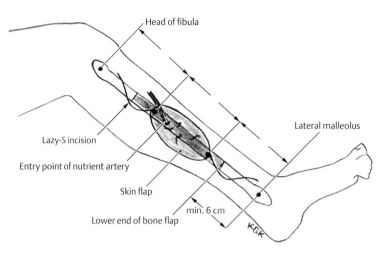

Fig. 9.3 Planning markings of the fibula flap.

Head of fibula

Lateral malleolus

Lazy-S incision

Entry point of nutrient artery

Skin flap

min. 6 cm

Lower end of bone flap

KGK

nerve lies in the direct neighborhood of the vascular pedicle and the deep peroneal nerve comes to the proximity of the latter as the interosseous septum is incised. These structures are respected and separated from the vascular pedicle.

During soft-tissue dissection underneath the skin island until the vascular pedicle, care is taken to include a thin cuff of the soleus and

flexor hallucis longus (posteriorly) and a cuff of the peroneal muscles (anteriorly) around the peroneal vessels by sharp dissection. This ensures the safe inclusion of the septocutaneous vessels that supply the skin flap.

Now the lazy-S incision proximal to the skin island is made and the fibula exposed. The proximal osteotomy is performed in a similar manner to the distal one. As the assistant posi-

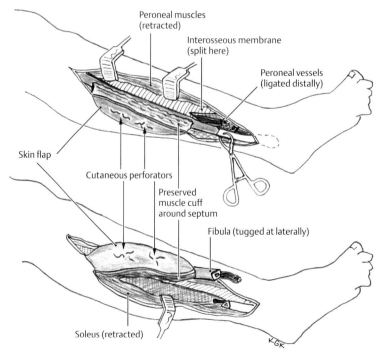

Fig. 9.4 Dissection of the fibula flap.

Peroneal muscles
(retracted)

Interosseous membrane
(split here)

Peroneal vessels
(ligated distally)

Skin flap

Cutaneous perforators

Preserved
muscle cuff
around septum

Fibula (tugged at laterally)

Soleus (retracted)

KGK

Fig. 9.5 The harvested fibula flap and some of its variations.

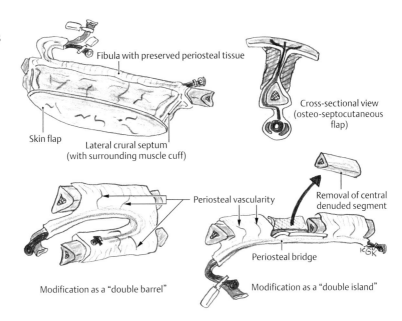

Fibula with preserved periosteal tissue

Cross-sectional view (osteo-septocutaneous flap)

Skin flap

Lateral crural septum (with surrounding muscle cuff)

Periosteal vascularity

Removal of central denuded segment

Periosteal bridge

Modification as a "double barrel"

Modification as a "double island"

tions the fibula flap in space, gently pulling it laterally, the operator follows the vascular pedicle to its origin from the posterior tibial vessels. Here the vessels are ligated, clipped, and divided.

It has been suggested that the lower end of the fibula be fixed with screws or a bone peg to prevent disruption of the ankle. However, I have not encountered postoperative problems, probably since I always leave enough bone in situ distally. The wound is closed primarily over a suction drain. Skin grafting may be necessary if a large skin flap is raised with the bone.

The fibula may be conveniently modified on the bench in various ways as the recipient site demands (**Fig. 9.5**). Osteotomies of different configuration (axial or transverse) and multitude may be performed as required, ensuring that the bridging periosteum is kept intact. The fibula has been modeled in double-barrelled fashion to augment height,[8] or split axially for achieving a suitable angle for mandibular reconstructions.[7] Recently we modified the bone as a "double-island," preserving a periosteal bridge between the islands, for the reconstruction of noncontiguous cervical vertebral bodies.[5] Both islands showed adequate bleeding after the completion of vascular anastomoses.

The vessels are approximately 2 mm in diameter and the pedicle is ~6–8 cm in length. If needs be, the pedicle may be lengthened by releasing it from the proximal part of the bone flap till the entry point of the nutrient artery. As a rule this maneuver is not necessary, for it may imperil the division of the nutrient artery, and besides, the length of pedicle already available (up to 8 cm) is usually ample.

Pitfalls

Failure to preserve enough fibular length in situ distally will cause unnecessary ankle instability. During early dissection it is important to separate and preserve the nerves that run in the vicinity of the vascular pedicle. Too thin a muscle cuff around the lateral crural septum or dissection too close to the septum might jeopardize the skin vascularity.

Finely controlled use of high-velocity instruments is called for in bench-modelling the bone flap. Here, it might be surprisingly quick and easy to disrupt the integrity of the vascular structures or the bridging periosteum.

A degree of peroneal weakness is to be expected during the initial period following harvesting of the fibula. This may be attributed to the separated muscle attachments and nerve manipulation. Usually the deficit is self-limiting, and rapid recuperation is observed in patients undergoing physical therapy.

References

1 *Gilbert A.* Free vascularized bone grafts. Int Surg 1981;66:27–31
2 *Taylor GI, Miller GD, Ham FJ.* The free vascularized bone graft. A clinical extension of microvascular techniques. Plast Reconstr Surg 1975;55(5):533–544
3 *Ceruso M, Falcone C, Innocenti M, Delcroix L, Capanna R, Manfrini M.* Skeletal reconstruction with a free vascularized fibula graft associated to bone allograft after resection of malignant bone tumor of limbs. Handchir Mikrochir Plast Chir 2001;33:277–282
4 *Judet H, Gilbert A.* Long-term results of free vascularized fibular grafting for femoral head necrosis. Clin Orthop Relat Res 2001; 386:114–119
5 *Krishnan KG, Müller A.* Ventral cervical fusion at multiple levels using free vascularized double-islanded fibula – a technical report and review of the relevant literature. Eur Spine J 2002;11(2):176–182
6 *Wei FC, Celik N, Chen HC, Cheng MH, Huang WC.* Combined anterolateral thigh flap and vascularized fibula osteoseptocutaneous flap in reconstruction of extensive composite mandibular defects. Plast Reconstr Surg 2002;109(1):45–52
7 *Guyot L, Richard O, Cheynet F,* et al. "Axial split osteotomy" of free fibular flaps for mandible reconstruction: preliminary results. Plast Reconstr Surg 2001; 108(2): 332–335
8 *Yajima H, Tamai S.* Twin-barrelled vascularized fibular grafting to the pelvis and lower extremity. Clin Orthop Relat Res 1994; 303:178–184
9 *Xijing H, Haopeng L, Liaosha J, Binshang L, Kunzheng W, Lvzhen M.* Functional development of the donor leg after vascularized fibula graft in childhood. J Pediatr Surg 2000;35(8):1226–1229
10 *Ad-El DD, Paizer A, Pidhortz C.* Bipedicled vascularized fibula flap for proximal humerus defect in a child. Plast Reconstr Surg 2001;107(1):155–157

Chapter 10
The Sural Flap

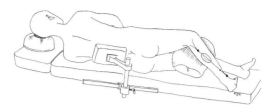

The superficial sensory nerves are, as a rule, accompanied by tiny vessels that also supply the overlying skin. The median superficial sural artery flap is based on this phenomenon. This flap was described as late as 1992 by Masquelet et al.,[1] when they presented an anatomical study and clinical application of skin island flaps based on the vessels accompanying the superficial sensory nerves of the leg. Later, Hasegawa et al.[2] refined the technique and showed that even large flaps survived when the deep fascia was included to the sural flap. Since then this flap has undergone several minor modifications to improve complete "take."[3] Reports, based on anatomical evidence, show the possibility of adding some of the underlying gastrocnemius muscle to the distally based flap.[4,5] The prominent qualities of the flap notwithstanding, a large series presented quite recently showed that the incidence of partial necrosis amounted to ~20% of cases.[6] Lately, I augmented the vascularity of the distally based flap by anastomosing the proximally divided median superficial sural vessels in the recipient site after rotating it and found that complete survival occurred. My experience is limited, but probably such an

Fig. 10.1 Patient positioning for the harvest of the superficial sural artery flap.

augmentation may be suggested if there is noticeably poor circulation in the flap after raising it.

The superficial sural artery may equally serve as a basis for proximally based rotation flaps.[7]

Preparation

As a rule this flap is used as an island flap to cover skin defects of the ipsilateral distal leg, ankle, or foot. Thus the patient may be profitably placed in the lateral decubitus, parkbench, or in the prone position, depending on the approach to the defect area (**Fig. 10.1**). A nonexsanguinating tourniquet is applied at the upper thigh, and the extremity is draped in a mobile manner, so as to vary the limb position intraoperatively as required.

Vascular Anatomy (Fig. 10.2)

The median superficial sural artery arises either directly from the popliteal artery (ca. 65% of

Fig. 10.2 Anatomical basis, planning markings, and dissection of the superficial sural artery flap.

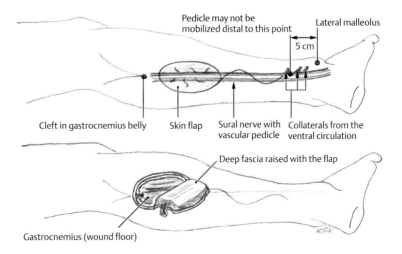

Pedicle may not be mobilized distal to this point

Lateral malleolus

5 cm

Cleft in gastrocnemius belly   Skin flap   Sural nerve with vascular pedicle   Collaterals from the ventral circulation

Deep fascia raised with the flap

Gastrocnemius (wound floor)

cases) or from the medial (ca. 20%) or lateral superficial sural arteries (ca. 8%). The artery runs posteriorly for 2–3 cm before joining the medial sural nerve, descending between the two heads of the gastrocnemius muscle. Then it courses alongside the sural nerve to the distal one-third of the leg, anastomosing with the supramalleolar branch of the peroneal artery and posterior tibial artery (ca. 5 cm above the lateral malleolus). Thus, in raising a distally based flap, it is important not to mobilize the flap too distally for fear of endangering these important anastomotic vessels. Usually, paired venae comitantes travel with this artery. Approximately four to eight fasciocutaneous perforators arising from the peroneal artery and venae comitantes follow the course of the posterior intermuscular septum to supply the crural fascia and skin. After penetrating the crural fascia, they give rise to several branches that communicate with adjacent perforators, forming an interconnecting vascular plexus on the crural fascia. The plexus extends from the posterior margin of the lateral malleolus to the superior part of the leg, thus practically a strip of skin overlying the course of the sural nerve can be raised on this pedicle.

Incisions and Dissection (Fig. 10.2)

A straight line is drawn connecting a point 1.5 cm posterior to the lateral malleolus and the cleft formed by the gastrocnemius muscle. This is the longitudinal axis of the sural nerve and the vascular pedicle. Further, a transverse line is marked 5 cm proximal to the lateral malleolus. This line marks the most distal point to which the pedicle may be mobilized. This flap can be located anywhere in the lower two-thirds of the posterior aspect of the leg according to need of pedicle length. The flap is then outlined and centered over the vascular pedicle drawn earlier according to the defect size.

An incision is made on the upper border of the flap, where the sural nerve as well as the vessels are identified at the midline, ligated, divided, and included with the flap. Incising the deep fascia superiorly, the dissection is performed in the subfascial plane, including the deep fascia with the flap. At this point one en-

counters musculocutaneous perforating vessels from the underlying gastrocnemius muscle. These are coagulated with fine bipolar cautery. At midcalf, the lazy-S incision is made and the nerve and vessels are identified, taking care not to skeletalize these structures. An ample amount of periareolar tissue, including the deep fascia, is left along with the pedicle. Now the tourniquet is deflated and the flap visibly attains color. The raised flap is then rotated to the defect to be reconstructed and sutured to the borders with tension-free sutures (**Fig. 10.3**).

I prefer to make a connecting skin incision to place the pedicle under direct vision rather than make a subcutaneous tunnel to pull the flap through. The donor site defect may be closed primarily.

If there is doubt about adequate perfusion, augmenting vascular anastomoses may be established between the previously divided proximal vessels and the vessels available at the recipient site. The vessels are approximately 1 mm in diameter and high magnification may be required for making the anastomoses.

Pitfalls

An absolute prerequisite for raising the superficial sural artery flap is an untouched lower third of the leg, at least. Usually, patients have been previously operated on in the lateral ankle region and may have developed sural nerve entrapment and corresponding pain. Not infrequently they would have received blocking injections of the sural nerve at various levels of the leg from their physicians. Eliciting this history is important and, in doubtful cases, a color-flow Doppler study may provide decisive information on vascular integrity. This is a relatively safe and reliable flap, as long as enough pedicle length is left in situ distally and enough periareolar tissue is raised with the pedicle. Pulling the distally based flap through a subcutaneous tunnel may cause stretch injury and/or kinking of the vessels. The patient is informed beforehand about the resulting sensory loss upon using this technique.

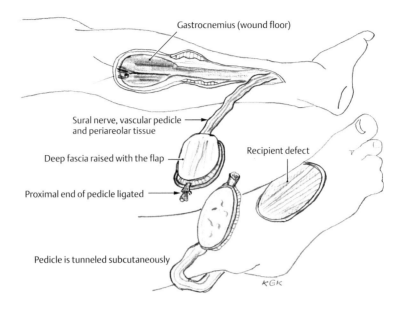

Fig. 10.3 The harvested superficial sural artery flap and an example of its application.

Gastrocnemius (wound floor)

Sural nerve, vascular pedicle and periareolar tissue

Recipient defect

Deep fascia raised with the flap

Proximal end of pedicle ligated

Pedicle is tunneled subcutaneously

References

1 *Masquelet AC, Romana MC, Wolf G.* Skin island flaps supplied by the vascular axis of the sensitive superficial nerves: anatomic study and clinical experience in the leg. Plast Reconstr Surg 1992;89(6):1115–1121

2 *Hasegawa M, Torii S, Katoh H, Esaki S.* The distally based superficial sural artery flap. Plast Reconstr Surg 1994;93(5):1012–1020

3 *Yilmaz M, Karatas O, Barutcu A.* The distally based superficial sural artery island flap. Plast Reconstr Surg 1998;102(7):2358–2367

4 *Le Fourn B, Caye N, Pannier M.* Distally based sural fasciomuscular flap: anatomic study and application for filling leg or foot defects. Plast Reconstr Surg 2001;107(1):67–72

5 *Mueller JE, Ilchmann T, Lowatscheff T.* The musculocutaneous sural artery flap for soft-tissue coverage after calcaneal fracture. Arch Orthop Trauma Surg 2001;121(6): 350–352

6 *Almeida MF, da Costa PR, Okawa RY.* Reverse-flow island sural flap. Plast Reconstr Surg 2002;109(2):583–591

7 *Karacalar A.* Axial bilobed flap based on the median and medial superficial sural arteries: a case report. Scand J Plast Reconstr Surg Hand Surg 2001;35(2):207–210

Chapter 11
The Dorsalis Pedis Flaps

The medial three toes, their metatarsals as well as the dorsal skin of the foot, are nourished by the dorsalis pedis artery. Thus any of these structures, separately or combined,[1] may be raised on the basis of the dorsalis pedis artery and the saphenous veins. Furthermore, it is possible to raise a skin flap based on the distal communications of the dorsalis pedis artery with the deep plantar arch.[2–4]

As early as 1967, Young[5] described reliable transfer of the second toe for thumb reconstruction in the Chinese language. However, it was not until two years later that the free toe transfer was reported in English.[6]

The dorsum of the foot offers thin, pliable, and reliably vascularized skin that also provides the option of using it as a neurosensate flap. Starting from narrow strips (for finger reconstruction) ending with almost the whole dorsum of the foot may be favorably transferred, based on the dorsalis pedis vessels, to meet different reconstructive challenges, especially of the hand. However, this flap has gained notoriety owing to the healing problems it leaves behind at its donor site.

Preparation

The positioning of the patient may be varied according to the approach to the recipient area, from supine to lateral decubitus. A strip of rolled soft gauze-cloth is used to grasp the first two toes in the manner shown in **Figure 11.1**

and the foot pulled to a more favorable plantar flexion. It is a good idea to apply a tourniquet to the thigh in a non-exsanguinating manner, so as to ease dissection of the subcutaneous veins.

Neurovascular Anatomy (Fig. 11.2)

The dorsalis pedis artery, the continuation of the anterior tibial artery, passes forward from the ankle-joint, lying beneath the retinaculum, along the tibial side of the dorsum of the foot to the proximal part of the first intermetatarsal space. Here it bifurcates into the first dorsal metatarsal and the deep plantar arteries, establishing communication with the deep plantar arch. At the level of the ankle this artery borders with the extensor hallucis longus from the tibial side, and with the first tendon of the extensor digitorum longus and the deep peroneal nerve from the fibular side. In a small minority of patients the dorsalis pedis artery may arise from the perforating branch of the deep peroneal artery. In these cases the flap pedicle remains short. The artery is accompanied by two comitant veins.

Infrequently the dorsal artery of the foot may be larger than usual, mostly to compensate for a deficient plantar artery; or its terminal branches to the toes may be absent, the toes then being supplied by the medial plantar. These anatomical variations are broadly classified under three types as shown in **Figure 11.2**. These variations do not play a role in raising the flap alone from the foot dorsum for free transfer. However, they have to be considered while planning a free toe transfer, or raising a distally based skin flap.

The greater and the lesser saphenous veins course along the tibial and the fibular aspects of the dorsal foot, respectively, receiving tributar-

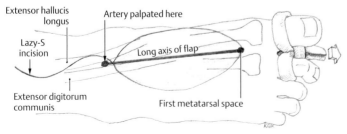

Fig. 11.1 Positioning and planning markings for the harvest of the dorsalis pedis flap.

Extensor hallucis longus

Artery palpated here

Lazy-S incision

Long axis of flap

Extensor digitorum communis

First metatarsal space

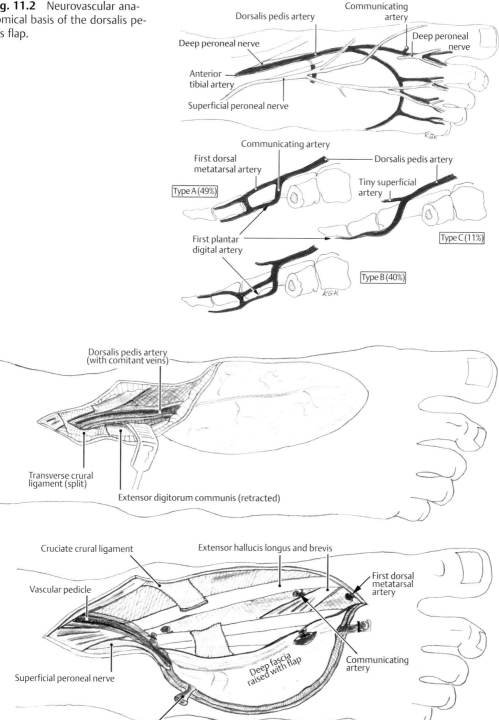

Fig. 11.2 Neurovascular anatomical basis of the dorsalis pedis flap.

Fig. 11.3 Dissection of the dorsalis pedis flap.

ies from a rich network of veins woven between them. These veins may additionally be anastomosed in the recipient site, in case the comitant veins offer insufficient venous drainage of the flap, which is extremely rare. On the other hand, pure venous flaps may be raised on the basis of the subcutaneous venous network described above.

Most of the dorsum of the foot is supplied by the superficial peroneal nerve. The first interdigital space is innervated by the deep peroneal nerve. The pulps of the medial three toes, which are mostly preferred for free transfer, receive sensory innervation through the digital branch of the medial plantar nerve (a musculocutaneous nerve).

Incisions and Dissection of the Dorsal Foot Flap (Figs. 11.1, 11.3)

The dorsalis pedis artery may be palpated at the dorsum of the ankle. A straight line drawn between this point and the first metatarsal space marks the long axis of the dorsal foot flap. A lazy-S incision is made at the proximal pole of the planned flap and the dorsalis pedis vessels as well as the superficial peroneal nerve identified. The tibial border of the flap including the deep fascia is then incised. At the distal pole of the flap the bifurcation of the dorsalis pedis

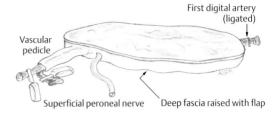

First digital artery (ligated)

Vascular pedicle

Superficial peroneal nerve   Deep fascia raised with flap

Fig. 11.4   The harvested dorsalis pedis flap.

vessels into the first metatarsal and the deep plantar are identified and ligated. The flap is then raised from medial to lateral, raising the deep fascia and the paratenon of the extensor tendons along with the skin. The cruciate crural ligament, which is one layer deeper to the deep fascia, is either incised and the pedicle vessels carefully taken out to be included with the flap, or a part of the ligament is included with the flap. The greater and the lesser saphenous veins, as well as the cutaneous nerve (if necessary) are also raised along with the flap (**Fig. 11.4**).

In raising small flaps, the donor defect may be stretched, after undermining the skin on both sides, and held to each other by applying large sutures till the end of the recipient operation. Usually the skin adapts to the created tension during this time. Direct closure may then be attempted at the end of the operation. A skin

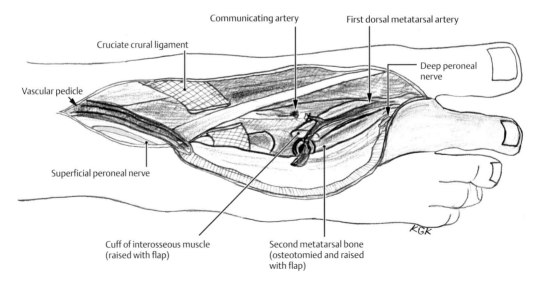

Communicating artery   First dorsal metatarsal artery

Cruciate crural ligament

Vascular pedicle

Deep peroneal nerve

Superficial peroneal nerve

Cuff of interosseous muscle (raised with flap)

Second metatarsal bone (osteotomied and raised with flap)

Fig. 11.5   Raising of the second toe based on the dorsalis artery.

Fig. 11.6 The harvested second toe and metacarpal bone based on the dorsalis pedis artery.

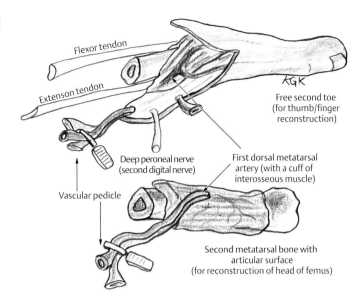

Flexor tendon

Extenson tendon

KGK

Free second toe
(for thumb/finger reconstruction)

Deep peroneal nerve
(second digital nerve)

First dorsal metatarsal artery (with a cuff of interosseous muscle)

Vascular pedicle

Second metatarsal bone with articular surface
(for reconstruction of head of femur)

graft becomes mandatory in raising larger flaps. Not infrequently one has to await and fight wound-healing problems at the donor site.

Incisions and Dissection for Raising the Toe (Figs. 11.5, 11.6)

When the toe is raised along with the dorsal foot flap, the dissection is proceeded as explained above with some modifications: a careful inspection of vessel ramifications at the first metatarsal space will reveal the presence or absence of the first dorsal metatarsal artery. If this artery is present, it is followed distally, revealing its branches, and the first or second toe or a combination of tissues (for instance, wrap-around fillet of the toes) is raised in a straightforward manner, raising the neighboring lumbrical muscles along with the flap. Cutting the second metatarsal bone at its middle third and hinging it provides more room for dissection in this area. In case the dorsal metatarsal artery is absent or too feeble, then the plantar arteries are carefully pursued through the space created by folding forward the osteotomied second metatarsal bone.

When raising of a toe or toe fillet alone is called for, then the incisions are made in a fishmouth fashion, running through the corresponding web spaces, and extended in a lazy-S shape both at the dorsal and plantar aspects of

the foot. The second metatarsal bone is osteotomied and raised with the flap, taking care to include a cuff of the lubrical muscles along with the pedicle vessels. Excessive bone and soft tissue of the flap are cut and discarded. Removal of a major part of the second metatarsal bone provides for the ray resection of the toe, enabling direct closure.

Pitfalls

In raising the dorsal foot flap, it is surprisingly easy to separate the pedicle vessels from the skin; thus the dissection should be cautiously performed in the subfascial plane, including the paratenon. Patients with peripheral vascular occlusion disease may prove to be poor candidates, since removing the dorsalis pedis artery might significantly compromise circulation. Wound dehiscence at the donor site may become troublesome. Despite its disadvantages the flap has won its place in hand reconstruction, due to the striking similarities exhibited between the extremities.

References

1 *Chang T-S, Wang W, Wu J-B.* Free transfer of the second toe combined with dorsalis pedis flap using microvascular technique for reconstruction of the thumb and other fingers. Ann Acad Med Singapore 1979;8:404–412

2 *Bharathwaj VS, Quaba AA*. The distally based islanded dorsal foot flap. Br J Plast Surg 1997;50(4):284–287

3 *Earley MJ, Milner RH*. A distally based first web flap in the foot. Br J Plast Surg 1989;42(5):507–511

4 *Pallua N, Di Benedetto G, Berger A*. Forefoot reconstruction by reversed island flap in diabetic patients. Plast Reconstr Surg 2000; 106(4):823–827

5 *Young TY*. Second toe free transfer for thumb reconstruction. Zhongua Wai Ke Za Zhi (Chinese J Surg) 1967;15:13

6 *Cobbett JR*. Free digital transfer. Report of a case of transfer of a great toe to replace an amputated thumb. J Bone Joint Surg Br 1969;51(4):677–679

Chapter 12
The Medial Plantar Flap

Since their description in 1979,[1] rotational skin flaps isolated on the medial plantar artery have been successfully used for covering defects of the plantar region, following the principle of reconstructing "like with like." As the vascular anatomical knowledge of the plantar skin gained depth,[2] this flap underwent several modifications to be used as a distally pedicled free flap[3–5] or, furthermore, as a small, free sensate flap for finger pulp reconstruction.[6,7]

Originally belonging to a nonweightbearing area of the foot, the skin of the medial plantar flap is relatively tough and rapidly adapts to new tasks at the recipient site; this especially applies to reconstructed plantar weightbearing areas. The possibility to raise the flap with the cutaneous nerves makes it an attractive option for finger pulp reconstruction. The donor site wound is directly closed and is nicely concealed in raising small flaps. The subcutaneous venous network is rich, offering the possibility of raising the skin as a venous flap.

Preparation

The patient is best positioned supine with his or her hip joint rotated externally and the knee flexed gently, so as to render the approach to the medial plantar region straightforward. A nonexsanguinating tourniquet is applied to the thigh.

Neurovascular Anatomy (Fig. 12.1)

The medial plantar artery is the medial branch of the posterior tibial artery, as the latter descends into the plantar region; the other branch is the lateral plantar artery. Being much smaller than the lateral branch, the medial plantar artery passes forward along the medial side of the foot, at first situated above the abductor hallucis, and then between it and the flexor digitorum brevis. At the base of the first metatarsal bone, where it is much diminished in size, it passes along the medial border of the first toe, anastomosing with the first dorsal metatarsal artery. Not infrequently, there is a connection to the deep plantar arterial arch through a communicating artery. The artery is accompanied by the medial plantar nerve that gives off sensory branches to the skin along its course. There are comitant veins accompanying the artery, in addition to the subcutaneous tributaries that run in the dorsal direction toward the great saphenous vein.

Incisions and Dissection (Figs. 12.2, 12.3)

The posterior tibial artery is palpated behind the medial malleolus and marked. The straight line connecting this point and plantar aspect of the first metatarsal space is divided into three equal parts. The border between the middle and distal thirds usually denotes the point

Fig. 12.1 The vascular anatomical basis of the plantar instep flap.

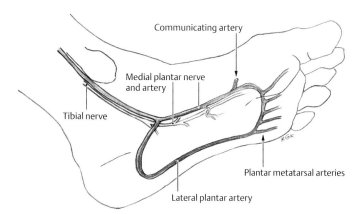

Communicating artery

Medial plantar nerve and artery

Tibial nerve

Lateral plantar artery

Plantar metatarsal arteries

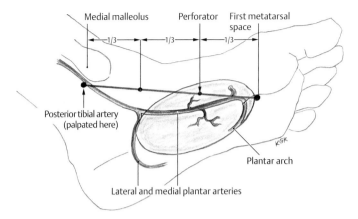

Fig. 12.2 Planning skin markings of the plantar instep flap.

Medial malleolus   Perforator   First metatarsal space

—1/3—→|←—1/3—→|←—1/3—→

Posterior tibial artery (palpated here)

Plantar arch

Lateral and medial plantar arteries

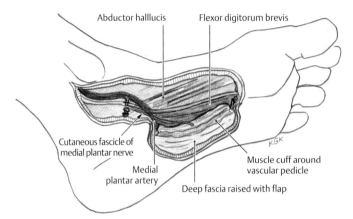

Fig. 12.3 Dissection of the plantar instep flap.

Abductor halllucis   Flexor digitorum brevis

Cutaneous fascicle of medial plantar nerve

Medial plantar artery

Muscle cuff around vascular pedicle

Deep fascia raised with flap

where a strong perforator is present. Thus this point should be the center of the flap. A curvilinear line drawn from the medial malleolus, running along the medial plantar region to the first metatarsal space, denotes the long axis of the flap.

The flap size (not exceeding 10 × 8 cm) is determined and marked. A lazy-S incision running from the proximal end of the flap to the medial malleolus allows the dissection of the vascular pedicle. This done, the medial flap incision is made till the deep fascia, which is raised along with the flap. Dissection is performed in the subfascial plane (and the plantar aponeurosis) till the vessels and the nerve are seen lying between the abductor hallucis and the flexor digitorum brevis muscles. A cuff of these muscles is raised along with the vessels. Usually one or two fascicles of the cutaneous nerve branch is

encountered during the dissection. These fascicles are followed to the medial plantar nerve. The latter may be internally neurolysed to add more length to the cutaneous nerve of the flap.

In raising a distally based flap two modifications are possible. (a) The medial plantar vessels along the proximal course are ligated and cut, and the flap is rotated based on its communications with the plantar arch and the dorsal arterial system as shown in **Figure 12.4**. (b) The medial plantar artery is followed to its origin from the posterior tibial, which gives off another branch here, namely the lateral plantar artery. Now the lateral plantar vessels are mobilized to a distance distally and the posterior tibial vessels are ligated well above their bifurcation. The resulting medial plantar skin flap is distally based on the lateral plantar arterial

Fig. 12.4 The harvested plantar instep flap and its variations.

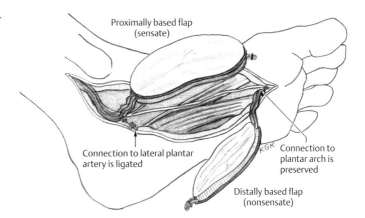

Proximally based flap (sensate)

Connection to lateral plantar artery is ligated

Connection to plantar arch is preserved

Distally based flap (nonsensate)

communication to the dorsalis pedis circulation. The flap is then cut and mobilized to the recipient area.[4] Skin grafting is necessary after raising large flaps.

Free flaps based on the medial plantar vessels pose great interest in hand and finger reconstruction. However, serial and long-term follow-up studies are lacking in the literature. As such reports become available, the medial plantar free flap might, owing to its low donor site morbidity, become a worthy competitor to the wrap-around toe fillet flaps.

> **Pitfalls**
>
> Careful dissection is called for, so that the vessels are not separated from the flap. It is a good idea to add a portion of the adductor hallucis and flexor digitorum brevis muscles along with the flap. The vessel diameter is approximately 1 mm. Dexterous technique is employed to achieve perfect anastomoses.

References

1 *Shanahan RE, Gingrass RP.* Medial plantar sensory flap for coverage of heel defects. Plast Reconstr Surg 1979;64:295–298

2 *Morrison WA, Crabb DM, O'Brien BM, Jenkins AL.* The instep of the foot as a fasciocutaneous island and as a free flap for heel defects. Plast Reconstr Surg 1983;72:56

3 *Bhandari PS, Sobti C.* Reverse flow instep island flap. Plast Reconstr Surg 1999; 103(7): 1986–1989

4 *Oberlin C, Accioli de Vasconcellos Z, Touam C.* Medial plantar flap based distally on the lateral plantar artery to cover a forefoot skin defect. Plast Reconstr Surg 2000; 106(4): 874–877

5 *Pallua N, Di Benedetto G, Berger A.* Forefoot reconstruction by reversed island flap in diabetic patients. Plast Reconstr Surg 2000; 106(4):823–827

6 *Koshima I, Urushibara K, Inagawa K, Hamasaki T, Moriguchi T.* Free medial plantar perforator flaps for the resurfacing of finger and foot defects. Plast Reconstr Surg 2001; 107(7):1753–1758

7 *Lee HB, Tark KC, Rah DK, Shin KS.* Pulp reconstruction of fingers with very small sensate medial plantar free flap. Plast Reconstr Surg 1998;101(4):999–1005

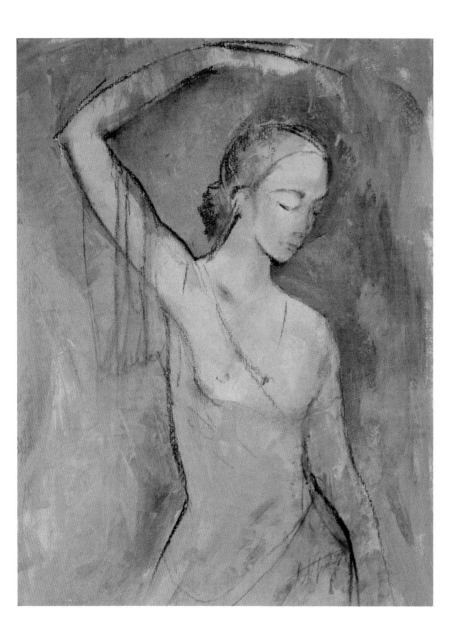

Part 3
Flaps of the Torso

Part 3
Flaps of the Torso

Both from historical and practical points of view, flaps of the torso play an important role in reconstructive microsurgery. Various flaps are possible that have well-defined and constant circulatory patterns; thus they are very reliable for reconstruction. The multitude of tissue components that may constitute flaps raised from the torso make them attractive for meeting various reconstructive challenges. Furthermore, the singularly excellent and predictable ramifications of vascular structures within the matter of such flaps enable diverse methods of bench modeling to fit the individual needs of the defects to be reconstructed.

In this part of the manual I have attempted to describe the techniques of harvesting eight free flaps and some of their modifications. Most of these flaps are from the integument and muscles; however, flaps such as the omentum and ileum can be raised from the abdominal cavity. When considering tissues for transplantation—autotransplantation or homotransplantation—harvesting of whole organs, such as the kidneys, liver, lungs, and the heart also falls into this category, all of which should be performed on small animals by the trainee in microvascular techniques. However, these operations fall outside the general scope of this manual, as does also the discipline of reconstructive microsurgery.

One further type of flap, which I have made no attempt to describe, is the so-called perforator flap: cutaneous territories can be successfully and reliably isolated based on perforating vessels from the underlying muscle structures. This is possible, as per description, from any surface of the body, provided the surgeon is ready to manipulate extremely small perforator vessels. This category of flaps is the next step in the learning curve of flap surgery.

Chapter 13
The Rectus Abdominis Muscle Flap

The rectus abdominis muscle as a free vascularized flap was first described by Pennington et al. in 1980.[1] According to the classification of Mathes and Nahai (see Chapter 21), the rectus abdominis muscle receives a type 3 vascular supply, with two dominant pedicles at either end of the muscle. This flap is useful for defects of moderate size requiring well-vascularized tissue, ranking between the gracilis and latissimus dorsi muscles in size. The rectus abdominis muscle measures ~30 cm × 10 cm in the adult in situ.

The rectus abdominis muscle can also be used as a reliable musculocutaneous flap. The skin island can be oriented in a variety of ways, depending on the defect size and orientation or donor scar preferences. The key to preserving the skin viability is to include the large perfora-tors from the rectus muscle, especially around the umbilicus.[2] If designed on an axis extending 45° and cephalad from the umbilicus, a skin paddle can extend to the anterior axillary line.[2]

The favorable anatomical location of the rectus abdominis muscle makes dissection convenient with the patient in a prone position, and enables a simultaneous two-team approach for coverage of defects on the anterior aspect of the body. The deep inferior epigastric vessels, based on which the muscle is raised as a free flap, amount to 2–4 mm in diameter, and the pedicle is usually 6–8 cm in length. A further 2–3 cm of pedicle length can be achieved by mobilization within the limits of the flap.

Preparation

Dissection is straightforward with the patient placed in the supine position. If reconstruction of the lower extremity is planned, as is usually the case, an angiography may be required to delineate donor vessels at the recipient site. Myorelaxants are administered to ease muscle retraction during flap harvest. Surface markings

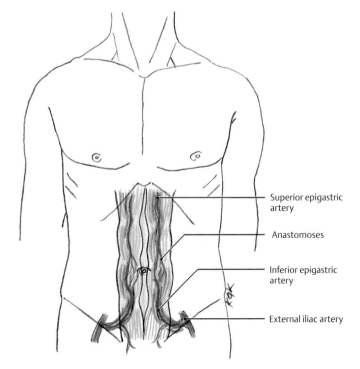

Fig. 13.1 The vascular anatomical basis of the rectus abdominis flap.

Superior epigastric artery

Anastomoses

Inferior epigastric artery

External iliac artery

Fig. 13.2 Planning markings of the rectus abdominis flap.

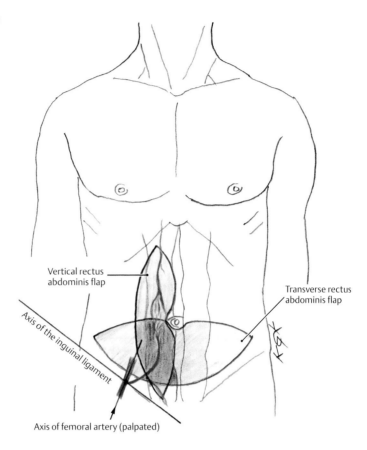

Vertical rectus abdominis flap

Transverse rectus abdominis flap

Axis of the inguinal ligament

Axis of femoral artery (palpated)

include the midline, the lateral muscle extent, and the iliofemoral axis, all of which can be palpated. The vascular pedicle originates ~1 cm above the inguinal ligament and enters the internal, lateral side of the muscle midway between the umbilicus and the pelvic crest.

Neurovascular Anatomy

The rectus abdominis is a broad, flat, paired muscle of the anterior abdominal wall. At their inferior origin, they are inserted by two (paired) tendinous attachments to the symphysis pubis and pubic crest. The muscle bellies run together cranially to insert onto the lower thoracic cartilages 5, 6, and 7 (**Fig. 13.1**). Ontogenetically, the rectus abdominis is formed from the fusion of the anterior mesodermal somites, the result of which appears in the specific fascial coalescences of the muscle: the rectus abdominis is ensheathed by fasciae arising from the external

and internal oblique, as well as the transverse musculature that forms both the anterior and posterior rectus sheaths, respectively. Above the linea arcuata, the anterior sheath is formed from the fascia of the external oblique and one of the two lamellae of the internal oblique muscles, whereas the posterior sheath consists of the deeper lamella of the internal oblique and the transversus abdominis muscles. Below the linea arcuata, the lamellae of the internal oblique and the transversus abdominis join together with the other fasciae and form the anterior sheath of the rectus. Thus the posterior aspect of the rectus abdominis muscle is devoid of fascial sheath beneath the linea arcuata (**Fig. 13.2**). After harvesting the muscle from this region, reinvestment is required,depending on the size of the defect, either by mobilizing lateral muscles or using synthetic meshes, for example, Gore-Tex, to prevent herniation of peritoneal contents.

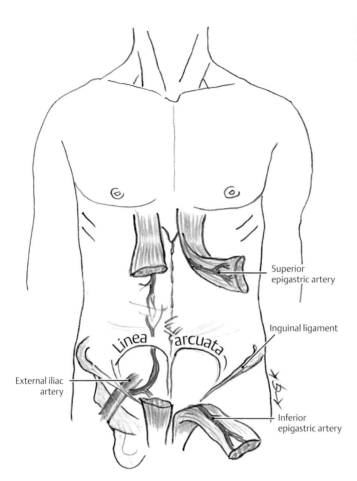

Fig. 13.3 Further internal and vascular anatomy of the rectus abdominis flap.

The rectus abdominis has a double polar blood supply that anastomoses in the central region of the muscle. The superior epigastric artery, a terminal branch of the internal mammary, enters at the junction of the xiphisternum and high diaphragmatic fiber insertion. The inferior epigastric artery arises from the external iliac artery below and behind the inguinal ligament to enter the posterior and lateral sheath at the level of the linea arcuata (**Fig. 13.3**). Each artery is accompanied by its venae comitantes, which drain into the internal mammary vein superiorly and the external iliac vein inferiorly. The deep inferior epigastric artery averages 2–4 mm in diameter and the superior 1–2 mm. The vasculature or the muscle can nourish large areas of the skin of the abdominal wall via perforators that communicate with the superficial vascular network. The most important of these perforators are located around the umbilicus. Both sensory and motor innervation arises from T7 to T12 segments.

Incisions and Dissection

The choice of the skin incision for a pure muscle flap depends on the amount of muscle required and the wishes of the patient regarding scar placement. A vertical paramedian incision is quick and efficient but leaves a noticeable scar. A transverse suprapubic incision with abdominal wall undermining gives good access to the lower muscle and the pedicle. Depending on the wishes of the patient, an abdominoplasty may be combined with muscle harvest. If a musculocutaneous flap is planned, an ellipse is drawn in a vertical or transverse orientation depending on the donor scar, as well as the re-

Fig. 13.4 Dissection and harvest of the rectus abdominis flap.

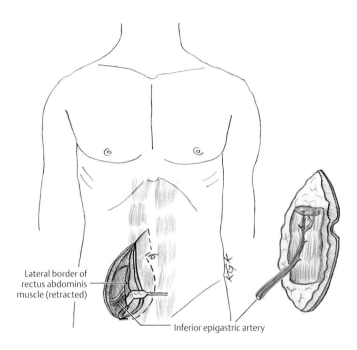

Lateral border of rectus abdominis muscle (retracted)

Inferior epigastric artery

quirements of the recipient site. Irrespective of design, care should be taken to include the large periumbilical perforators.

The lateral skin incisions in approximation to the vascular pedicle are made first. The muscle sheath attachments are divided at the lateral border of the muscle. Dissection below, and lateral to, the muscle will expose the interior epigastric vessels that are seen to enter the deep portion of the muscle at the level of the linea arcuata (**Fig. 13.4**). Once the vessels are isolated, the rest of the skin incisions are completed. The muscle sheath attachments at the linea alba are divided medially and the lateral sheath is incised, taking care to ligate segmental vessels. The segmental nerves may be preserved, if functional muscle transfer is preferred. The dimension of the muscle harvested depends on the requirements of the recipient site. The muscle is incised at its cranial end accordingly. Later, the caudal end is incised and the muscle is isolated on its vascular pedicle, the deep inferior epigastric vessels, which may be traced to their origin from the external iliac vessels.

The vascular pedicle is usually 6–8 cm long. The vessels have diameters of ~2–4 mm. Sometimes, instead of venae comitantes, a conjoint vein may be found, which is 4–5 mm in diameter.

Pitfalls

Disadvantages of the free rectus abdominis flap are few. A vertical abdominal scar will be found annoying. Scarring can be minimized by using a low transverse incision, combined with an abdominoplasty. Sometimes, previous abdominal surgery may have interfered with the vascular pedicle. The muscle can be transplanted on its superior pedicle if the inferior one has been destroyed; however, the superior epigastric vessels are much smaller. With a preserved anterior rectus sheath (in case of a pure muscle flap), abdominal herniation is of minimal concern. With removal of the anterior sheath with the musculocutaneous flap, the risk of herniation is greater, requiring reinvestment using mobilized lateral muscles or a Gore-Tex synthetic mesh substitute. Obese patients are poor candidates for a musculocutaneous flap because of the bulk of adipose tissue and unreliable perforators. Not seldom in such cases will a secondary debulking surgery be required at the recipient area. The segmental nerve supply limits the use of rectus abdominis as a functional muscle transplant; other muscle flaps may be found more reliable in this respect.

References

1 *Pennington DG, Lai MF, Pelly AD.* The rectus abdominis myocutaneous free flap. Br J Plast Surg 1980;33:277–282

2 *Boyd JB, Taylor GI, Corlett R.* The vascular territories of the superior epigastric and inferior epigastric systems. Plast Reconstr Surg 1984; 73:1–16

Chapter 14
The Groin Flap

Historically, the groin flap was one of the first cutaneous flaps to be moved from the experimental and anatomy laboratory into the clinic.[1-3]

The free groin flap is seldom indicated in today's practice, since a variety of more reliable free skin flaps have come to replace it. However, a groin flap medially attached on a cutaneous pedicle is still preferred by many for resurfacing defects of the hand dorsum in a two-staged procedure.[2,4] More often, highly vascularized muscle flaps are indicated, since they are more resistant to infection than subcutaneous fat tissue. However, there are also reports to the contrary.[5] The major advantage of the groin flap is its inconspicuous linear scar at the donor area. The anatomical location is favorable, making dissection convenient in the supine patient and enabling a two-team approach for coverage of defects on the anterior aspect of the body. The vascular pedicle of the free groin flap, consisting of the superficial circumflex iliac artery and comitant veins, is short, feeble, and demonstrates a high level of inconsistency, disadvantages that had led to the development of other cutaneous free flaps with more consistent vascular pedicles. In spite of all the drawbacks, groin flaps are still successfully used by various surgical subspecialties; thus their description is called for. Some authors have developed a perforator flap based on the superficial circumflex iliac vessels.[5]

Preparation

The patient is placed in the supine position. If a long flap is preferred, a stack of towels is placed under the buttock of the donor side to elevate the area to ease posterior dissection. The longitudinal axis of the flap parallels the inguinal ligament (**Fig. 14.1**). Cutaneous flaps can extend beyond the iliac crest posteriorly with dimensions of up to 30 cm or more in length and

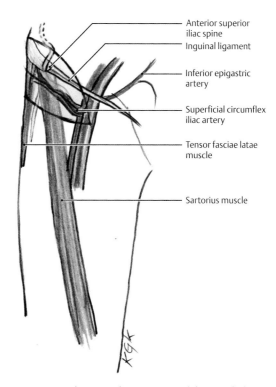

Anterior superior iliac spine

Inguinal ligament

Inferior epigastric artery

Superficial circumflex iliac artery

Tensor fasciae latae muscle

Sartorius muscle

Fig. 14.1 The vascular anatomical basis of the groin flap.

15 cm in width. Preoperative Doppler examination will prove useful in locating and following the course of the superficial circumflex iliac vessels. When preoperative angiography of the recipient site is mandated, for example, lower extremity, the radiologist should be made aware of the side-preference of the groin flap, so that a femoral artery puncture on this side is avoided.

Neurovascular Anatomy

The skin overlying the inguinal area extending beyond the borders of the anterior superior iliac spine can be isolated on the superficial circumflex iliac artery, originating directly from the femoral artery ~1 cm caudal to the inguinal ligament, and its venae comitantes (**Fig. 14.2**). As already mentioned, the anatomy of these vessels is widely variable. Venous drainage of the groin flap is accomplished not only by comitant veins, but also by direct cutaneous veins draining into the greater saphenous system. The superficial veins are often 2 mm or more in

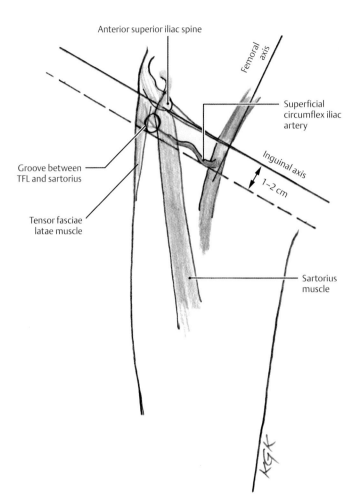

Anterior superior iliac spine

femoral axis

Superficial circumflex iliac artery

Inguinal axis

1~2 cm

Groove between TFL and sartorius

Tensor fasciae latae muscle

Sartorius muscle

Fig. 14.2 Planning markings of the groin flap. TFL, tensor fasciae latae.

diameter and can drain the entire groin flap satisfactorily, enabling easier connection in comparison to the venae comitantes of the superficial circumflex iliac artery which are usually much smaller. One further variation of the vascularity is seen with vessels accompanying the lateral femoral cutaneous nerve, which anastomose freely with the superficial circumflex iliac system. The groove between the tensor fasciae latae and the sartorius muscle can be palpated: the lateral femoral cutaneous nerve pierces the deep fascia approximately at this point.

Sensory innervation of the groin area is via a tiny branch of the T12 segmental nerve. However, a medial branch of the lateral femoral cutaneous nerve can also be observed. It is often difficult to identify and isolate cutaneous nerves of the groin flap in obese individuals.

Incisions and Dissection

Skin incisions are placed at the tip of the flap (laterally). It is often possible to identify and harvest the cutaneous nerve (terminal branch of the T12 segmental nerve) entering the lateral aspect of the flap in slender patients; however this might prove to be a tedious task in obese individuals. The nerve can usually be identified ~3–5 cm below the posterior iliac spine, where it pierces the deep fascia of the lateral thigh (**Fig. 14.3**). The nerve may be traced proximally to gain additional length. Once this nerve has been identified and transected, the flap can be elevated quickly to the level of the anterior superior iliac spine in a plane above the deep fascia without worry of injuring any key structures. The deep fascia overlying the sartorius

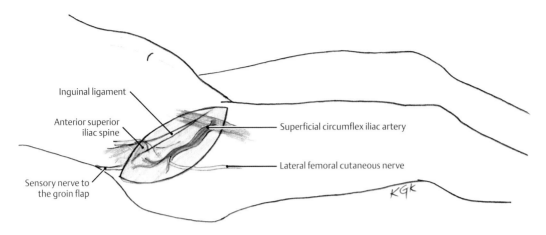

Fig. 14.3   Positioning and geometrical planning of the groin flap.

muscle is incised sharply and included with the flap to permit trapping of cutaneous microvessels coming from the superficial circumflex iliac system. Contrary to dissection of free muscle flaps, the groin flap here is raised simultaneously both in its superior and inferior aspects. As dissection proceeds, one can usually visualize the superficial circumflex iliac vessels on the under surface of the fascia (**Fig. 14.4**). Incision of the deep fascia overlying the sartorius muscle is now completed, so as to visualize deep vascular branches that pierce the deep fascia to nourish the sartorius muscle; these are coagulated with low-voltage bipolar cautery

forceps and transected. The dissection is carried across the floor of the femoral triangle to the lateral edge of the femoral sheath to identify the origin of the superficial circumflex iliac artery from the femoral artery. In completing the skin incisions on the medial aspect of the flap, the superficial veins are identified, followed to the saphenous system, transected there, and raised with the free flap.

The vascular pedicle is usually very short, ranging from 3 to 5 cm in length. The vessels have diameters of ~1–1.5 mm. Superficial draining veins may have a slightly larger diameter (ca. 2 mm).

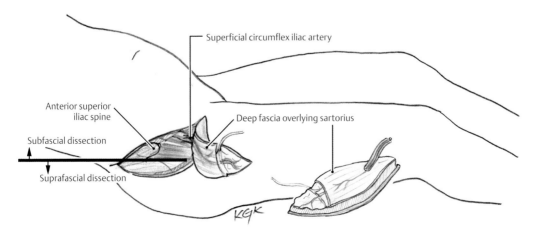

Fig. 14.4   Dissection and harvest of the groin flap.

Pitfalls

As already mentioned, the vascular anatomy of the groin flap is widely variable, keeping surprises in store. The vascular pedicle is short. In obese individuals, the subcutaneous fat tissue is a major hindrance at the recipient area, which calls for a secondary debulking surgery at a later stage. Some of the secondary flap-thinning surgery might have drastic effects. Thus, in my opinion, the free groin flap should be reserved for cases where other options are unavailable. However, utilizing the medially pedicled groin flap for reconstruction of defects of the dorsum of the hand in a two-staged procedure is a very reliable surgical procedure, the disadvantage being the two-staged nature of this reconstruction.

References

1 *McGregor IA, Jackson IT.* The groin flap. Br J Plast Surg 1972;25(1):3–16

2 *Milton SH.* The effect of delay on survival of experimental pedicle skin flap. Br J Plast Surg 1969;22:244–252

3 *Smith PJ, Foley B, McGregor IA, Jackson IT.* The anatomical basis of the groin flap. Plast Reconstr Surg 1972;49(1):41–47

4 *Goodstein WA, Buncke HJ* Jr. Patterns of vascular anastomosis vs. success of free groin flap transfer. Plast Reconstr Surg 1979;64:37–40

5 *Hsu WM, Chao WN, Yang C,* et al. Evolution of the free groin flap: the superficial circumflex iliac artery perforator flap. Plast Reconstr Surg 2007;119(5):1491–1498

Chapter 15
The Free Iliac Crest Bone Flap

The free vascularized bone flap from the iliac crest, based on the deep circumflex iliac vessels, was first described by Taylor et al. in 1975.[1] The tricortical bone structure offers both cortical and spongiosa components; thus bone healing and fusion at the donor area are excellent, surpassing other bone flaps. Owing to its naturally persistent curvature, this flap is popular among maxillofacial surgeons for reconstruction of mandibular defects. Its further use for vascularized reconstruction of head of femur in atresia has been stressed.[2] Combined with the superficial circumflex iliac system, corresponding to the groin flap, this bone graft has become firmly established as a reliable technique for reconstructing a large bone gap, especially if an associated soft-tissue defect is present. However, for tubular bone reconstruction, the iliac crest bone flap ranks second to the free fibula, which undisputedly offers a sturdier skeletal support to use in reconstruction of weightbearing bones.

Advantages of the groin flap are also applicable to the free iliac crest bone flap: (a) inconspicuous linear scar at the donor area; (b) the loss of the bony contour of the hip is not apparent; and (c) a favorable anatomical location that offers convenient dissection and enables a two-team approach. The vascular pedicle of the free iliac crest bone flap consists of the deep circumflex iliac vessels, which is more robust and reliable than the superficial circumflex iliac vessel system.

Preparation

The patient is placed in the supine position. If a long skin component of an osseocutaneous flap is planned, a stack of towels is placed under the buttock of the donor side to elevate the area to ease posterior dissection. The longitudinal axis of the flap lies parallel to the inguinal ligament (**Fig. 15.1**). As in preparing for the groin flap, any preoperative angiography should avoid

puncture of the femoral artery on the side of the planned iliac crest flap. Failure to do so will make dissection of the vascular pedicle of the flap, which is concealed in hematoma, unpleasant.

Neurovascular Anatomy

The crest of the ilium is nourished around the majority of its circumference by microvessels perforating the medial cortex just below its inner lip, as well as a rich network of periosteal vessels that drape the iliac fossa. These nutrient arteries arise from the deep circumflex iliac artery. This pattern of double vascular nourishment enables the removal of the outer cortex or modeling by multiple osteotomies, still without compromising the blood supply. The deep circumferential iliac vessels arise from the external iliac vessels, then traverse the deep fascia overlying the iliopsoas muscle, lining the inner rim close to the iliac crest as it provides the direct nutrient vessels as well as the periosteal vessels (**Fig. 15.1**).

As it courses the inner lip of the iliac crest, the deep circumflex iliac artery also gives off branches to the internal and external oblique muscles of the abdomen, and consequently perforator branches supply the skin overlying this area. Thus, the osteocutaneous flap can either include an area of skin attached to the bone through a cuff of the abdominal muscles of this region, or it may include the superficial circumflex iliac system, which also freely anastomoses with the deep system.

Incisions and Dissection

In raising an osteocutaneous flap, the integumentary portion of the flap is centered over the iliac crest, with its medial portion extending to the femoral vessels and its posterior extending maximally 8–10 cm behind the anterior superior iliac spine. The origin of the vascular pedicle is dissected first, before continuing to the flap as follows: through the medial skin incision, the femoral artery is exposed and followed proximally until the superficial circumflex iliac artery is found. The inguinal ligament is freed from attachments and retracted superi-

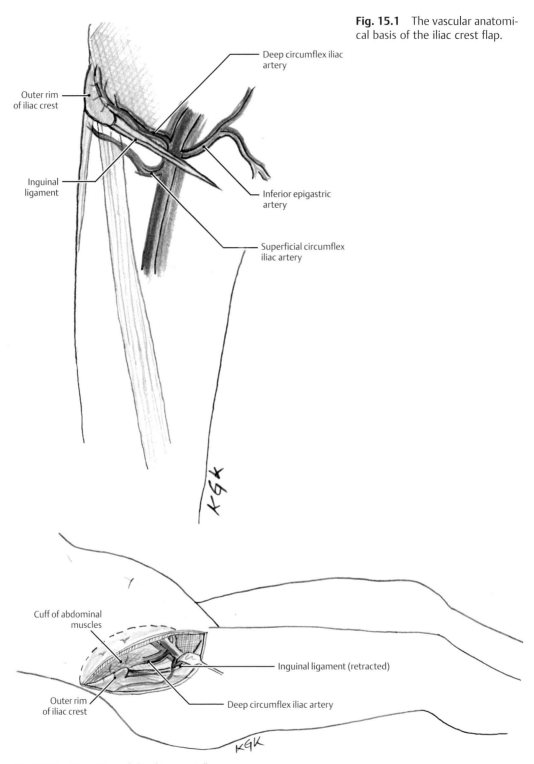

Fig. 15.1 The vascular anatomical basis of the iliac crest flap.

Deep circumflex iliac artery

Outer rim of iliac crest

Inguinal ligament

Inferior epigastric artery

Superficial circumflex iliac artery

Cuff of abdominal muscles

Inguinal ligament (retracted)

Outer rim of iliac crest

Deep circumflex iliac artery

Fig. 15.2   Dissection of the iliac crest flap.

orly until the deep circumflex iliac artery is encountered coming off the anterolateral or lateral aspect of the external iliac artery, usually 2 cm deep within the inguinal ligament (**Fig. 15.2**). The deep inferior epigastric artery, used in the rectus abdominis flap, has its origin medially at this same level. Next the venae comitantes of the deep circumflex iliac system are isolated.

The skin incision along the upper border of the planned osteocutaneous flap is now completed to enhance exposure. The incision extends in depth through the external oblique, internal oblique, and transversalis muscles of the abdominal wall to include the deep circumflex iliac vessels within the cuff. The island of skin should be carefully left attached to the muscle cuff on the inner rim of the iliac crest to prevent shearing off the delicate cutaneous perforators. Now the inferior skin incision of the island is completed and continued to the depth through the deep fascia overlying the tensor fasciae latae and gluteal muscles. From the inferior aspect of dissection, the iliac crest is released from the attachments of these above-mentioned muscles. Then the osteotomy of the iliac crest is performed, ensuring preservation of the muscle cuff around the deep circumflex

iliac vessels and the flimsy skin perforators (**Fig. 15.3**). Attention is now diverted to the anteromedial aspect to complete the dissection, taking care to preserve the superficial circumflex iliac vessels as they enter the cutaneous portion of the flap. Since these vessels were primarily dissected medially, dissection is performed from medial to lateral to complete the flap dissection. The vessels are ligated at their origin from the external iliac vessels, and the flap is harvested.

At the recipient site, after microvascular anastomoses of the deep circumflex vessels are completed, the adequacy of perfusion of the skin component is carefully observed. With inadequate connection between the deep and superficial vascular systems, perfusion of the cutaneous portion will fail. If this happens, augmenting anastomoses are required between the superficial circumflex iliac artery and another donor artery at the recipient site. Sometimes, an end-to-side anastomosis is established on the bench between the superficial and deep circumflex iliac arteries, before transplanting the flap.

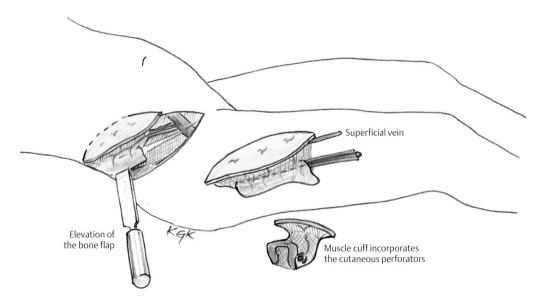

Superficial vein

Elevation of the bone flap

KGK

Muscle cuff incorporates the cutaneous perforators

Fig. 15.3 Harvest of the iliac crest flap.

Pitfalls

There are no major pitfalls involved in harvesting the iliac crest free flap. However, an osteocutaneous flap might show irregularities, requiring microvascular augmentation via additional anastomoses. Furthermore, the dissection of the vascular pedicle in the depth is a tedious manipulation. Caution should be exercised when using high-power instrumentation, such as the oscillating saw, so as to prevent microvascular accidents.

References

1 *Taylor GI, Miller GD, Ham FJ*. The free vascularized bone graft. A clinical extension of microvascular techniques. Plast Reconstr Surg 1975;55:533–544

2 *Marti RK, Schueller HM, van Steijn MJ*. Superolateral bone grafting for acetabular deficiency in primary total hip replacement and revision. J Bone Joint Surg Br 1994;76:728–734

Chapter 16
The Serratus Anterior Muscle Flap

The serratus anterior muscle as a free vascularized flap was described by Takayanagi et al.[1] It is a large muscle arising from the 1st to 9th ribs. Usually the lower three slips, which attach themselves to the 7th, 8th, and 9th ribs, are easily accessible and have a relatively independent innervation and vascularity; thus these slips are best suited for free transfer. Depending on the size of the recipient defect, the number of muscle slips to be transferred is determined.[2] The serratus anterior muscle is innervated by the relatively long and isolated long thoracic nerve. Additionally, owing to its specific anatomical configuration, which is easily modified as required without interrupting its neurovascular integrity, the muscle is well suited for dynamic reanimation of the paralyzed face.[3] The upper slips of the serratus anterior receive vascular supply from the long thoracic artery and comitant veins, whereas the lower slips are supplied by a branch to serratus anterior arising from the thoracodorsal trunk. Accordingly the muscle is classified as Mathes and Nahai type 3 (see Chapter 21).

The serratus anterior is useful for reconstruction of defects of small to moderate configuration requiring well vascularized tissue. Additionally a large skin component can be raised based on the perforating vessels. Furthermore, the attachment of the serratus anterior to the underlyng rib may be carefully preserved and the flap raised may include a bone component.

Preparation

Patient positioning depends on the recipient site: when the flap is used to reconstruct defects of the head and neck, the patient is positioned laterally, with the recipient site facing upward; when the muscle flap is used for facial reanimation, the donor side of the torso is padded, so as to allow posterior undermining and dissection. In both cases, the arm of the donor side is abducted and placed on an appropriately positioned armrest; the surgeon harvesting the flap stands between the outstretched arm and the torso, or at the back of the laterally placed patient. Muscle relaxing agents help dissection in the depth by easing retraction of adjacent muscles; they may be applied from the beginning in structural reconstructions or, in case of a functional muscle transfer, soon after the neural pedicle of the muscle has been identified and slung in a vessel loop.

Neurovascular Anatomy

The free serratus anterior muscle flap, musculocutaneous or osteomusculocutaneous flaps, usually includes the lower slips of the muscle. The entire serratus anterior muscle, starting from the 1st rib and ending with the 9th rib, has a dual vascular supply: the upper portion of the serratus is nourished by the lateral or long thoracic artery, located more anteriorly, which branches off the second part of the axillary artery under the pectoralis minor muscle; whereas the lower slips covering the 6th to 9th ribs are supplied by an arterial branch arising from the thoracodorsal artery of the subscapular arterial system (**Fig. 16.1**). The innervation of the serratus anterior muscle is by means of the long thoracic nerve, which courses down subfascially and somewhat anterior to the vascular pedicle, approximately on the mid surface of the muscle. The lower part of the serratus (lower three slips) has a well-defined nerve and blood supply, which enables it to be isolated as a transferable unit. The cutaneous territory of the serratus anterior musculocutaneous flap borders or overlaps with that of the latissimus dorsi muscle, and is located mainly between the anterior and middle axillary lines, with the possibility of extension on either side, as requirement dictates (**Fig. 16.2**).

Incisions and Dissection

The anterior and middle axillary lines are drawn. The anterior border of the latissimus dorsi muscle is palpated and marked, as are the 7th to 9th ribs. The muscular interdigitating mass covering these ribs represents the serratus

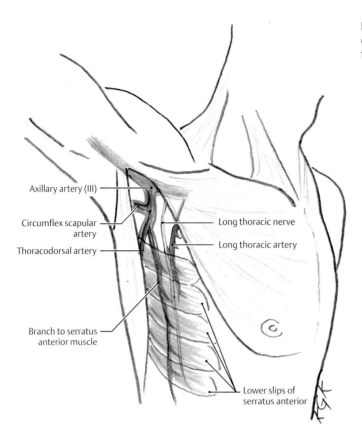

Fig. 16.1 The vascular anatomical basis of the serratus anterior flap.

Labels in figure:
- Axillary artery (III)
- Circumflex scapular artery
- Thoracodorsal artery
- Branch to serratus anterior muscle
- Long thoracic nerve
- Long thoracic artery
- Lower slips of serratus anterior

anterior muscle to be harvested. In raising a musculocutaneous flap, an elliptical skin area directly overlying the muscle slips is drawn.

The initial approach to the neurovascular pedicle is very much identical to raising the latissimus dorsi flap: the anterior border of the cutaneous island is incised first, extending it as necessary curving posteriorly and superiorly to enter the axilla. The vascular pedicle is easily visualized with the anterior border of the latissimus dorsi retracted. Often, the vessels to the upper slips of the serratus anterior (long thoracic artery, which springs directly from the axillary artery) is mistaken for the vascular pedicle of the planned flap, which consists of the three to five lower slips of the muscle. The blood supply here is achieved from the continuation of the subscapular–thoracodorsal pool. This is visualized with a retracted anterior border of the latissimus dorsi muscle lying on the serratus anterior muscle. There might be several branches that enter adjacent muscles;

these are divided between ligating clips. Proximally, once the vascular pedicle has been identified and slung with a vessel loop, the thoracodorsal artery to the latissimus dorsi muscle can be sacrificed and the dissection may be extended into the axilla to gain an extremely long vascular pedicle (**Fig. 16.3**). As a rule, this sacrifice is not necessary, since the vascular pedicle from the point of its entry into the serratus anterior muscle to its branching from the thoracodorsal artery is ~10 cm in length, which fulfils the requirements of any usual reconstruction.

The neural pedicle (the long thoracic nerve) is identified anterior to the vessels and is usually found underneath the fascia covering the serratus anterior muscle. As one proceeds with raising the neural pedicle, care is taken to preserve innervation to the slips of the serratus anterior left back in situ. Failure to do so will result in postoperative scapula alata. If a long nerve pedicle is required, as in the case of a

Fig. 16.2 Planning markings of the serratus anterior flap.

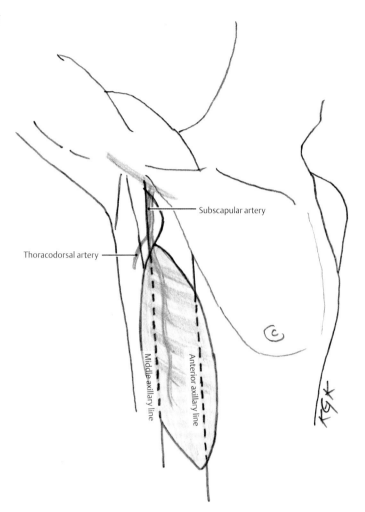

Subscapular artery

Thoracodorsal artery

Middle axillary line

Anterior axillary line

one-staged facial reanimation, it is perhaps wise to insert a sural nerve graft to reinnervate the remaining slips of the serratus anterior.

Once the neurovascular pedicle has been identified, dissected, and slung with a vessel loop, the rest of the flap harvesting steps are completed briskly as follows. The posterior skin incision is completed, and the lower border of the muscle flap is opened with monopolar cautery to reach the plane underneath (above the ribs). From then on, blunt digital dissection is performed to elevate the planned flap, being careful to avoid tension on the neurovascular pedicle (**Fig. 16.4**). Once the planned slips of the flap have been separated, the muscle can be detached from the rib cage with sharp dissection.

Perforating vessels entering the intercostal microvascular system can be observed as one proceeds with elevation of the flap from the underlying ribs. These are appropriately coagulated using a bipolar cautery, or ligated using clips. As a variation, when a bone component is required in reconstruction, these perforators are preserved and the 8th or 9th ribs, or both, are osteotomied anteriorly and posteriorly to the muscle flap and elevated along with the flap. In such a configuration, the rib can survive on the blood supply it receives via the muscle perforators (**Fig. 16.5**).

The vascular pedicle is usually approximately 8–10 cm in length, and may be lengthened during harvest by sacrificing the thoraco-

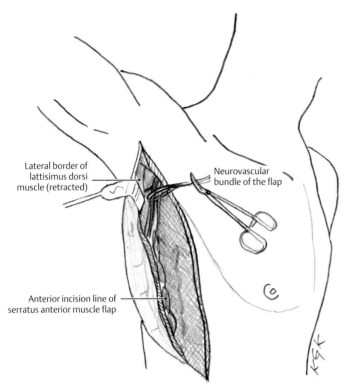

Fig. 16.3 Dissection of the serratus anterior flap.

Lateral border of
lattisimus dorsi
muscle (retracted)

Neurovascular
bundle of the flap

Anterior incision line of
serratus anterior muscle flap

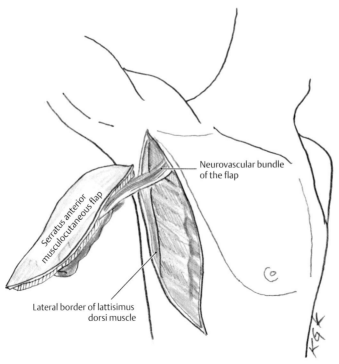

Fig. 16.4 Harvest of the serratus anterior flap.

Serratus anterior
musculocutaneous flap

Neurovascular bundle
of the flap

Lateral border of lattisimus
dorsi muscle

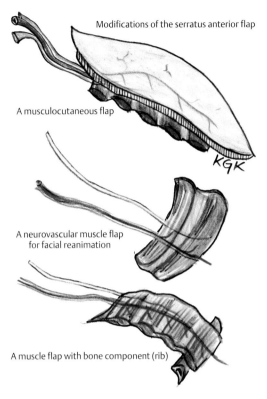

Modifications of the serratus anterior flap

A musculocutaneous flap

KGK

A neurovascular muscle flap
for facial reanimation

A muscle flap with bone component (rib)

Fig. 16.5   Some variations of the serratus anterior flap.

dorsal artery and carrying the dissection up into the subscapular system. The vessels have diameters of ~1.5–2 mm at their origin from the thoracodorsal system.

Pitfalls

Usually the serratus anterior is a reliable and spendable muscle flap that does not create subsequent sequelae at the donor site. However, failure to preserve innervation to the slips of the serratus anterior muscle left back in situ will cause winging of the scapula, which might require secondary reconstruction.

References

1 *Takayanagi S, Tsukie T.* Free serratus anterior muscle and musculocutaneous flaps. Ann Plast Surg 1982;8:277–283
2 *Whitney TM, Bunke HJ, Alpert BS, Bunke GM, Lineaweaver WC.* The serratus anterior free muscle flap: experience with 100 consecutive cases. Plast Reconstr Surg 1990;86:481–490
3 *Ueda K, Harii K, Yamada A.* Free vascularized double muscle transplantation for the treatment of facial paralysis. Plast Reconstr Surg 1995;95:1288–1296

Chapter 17
The Latissimus Dorsi Muscle Flap

The latissimus dorsi muscle is perhaps the most reliable and most versatile free flap available in the armamentarium of the reconstructive surgeon. It is also the largest unit available for transfer. The flat and fanlike geometry of the muscle allows its transformation by trimming, folding, rolling etc., to fit soft-tissue defects of practically any configuration, size, and shape. Furthermore, the posterior parts of the lower three ribs can be raised based on the vascular pedicle of the latissimus dorsi flap, dramatically increasing its versatility. Because of its well-defined innervation, the latissimus dorsi can be transplanted as a functional motor unit for purposes of dynamic reanimation of extremities; or, after thinning and appropriate tailoring, can also be used in reanimation of facial paralyses.

Transplantation of the noninnervated latissimus dorsi muscle flap for restoring structural incongruities has an additional advantage: the muscle fills the defect (obliterating dead spaces) and takes its shape with the passage of time, just as a fluid takes the shape of the vessel into which it is poured. By virtue of denervation the muscle mass atrophies quickly after transfer, restoring the contour of the recipient site. In my experience of using tailored latissimus dorsi muscle for scalp reconstruction in chronic wound healing problems after multiple neurocranial surgical procedures (12 cases), as well as anterior skull base reconstructions in chronic intractable frontobasal cerebrospinal fluid leakage (5 cases), the initially apparent muscle bulk disappeared to leave a pliable contour of the scalp or the skull base, respectively, within 2 weeks after transplantation. These were both clinically visible and could be documented with magnetic resonance imaging studies.

The latissimus dorsi muscle as a free vascularized muscle flap was perhaps first described by Maxwell et al. in 1978.[1] The vascular supply of the latissimus dorsi in situ is mainly through the subscapular–thoracodorsal axis, based on which it is isolated for transfer, and secondarily through multiple minor segmental branches; this comes under type 5 according to the Mathes and Nahai Classification (see Chapter 21). Further application of the latissimus dorsi muscle lies in its availability as a strong motor unit for unipolar or bipolar transfers in cases of irreparable upper brachial plexus lesions. Its constancy of anatomy, relative ease of harvest, negligible donor site morbidity, and paramount reliability make the free latissimus dorsi flap an indispensible tool in the armamentarium of any surgical subspecialty.

Preparation

Patient positioning on the lateral decubitus position with the arm abducted and placed on an armrest. Angiography for delineation of vessels at the recipient site may be required in patients with vascular occlusive diseases or in postradiation status. Muscle relaxants may be administered for easier muscle retraction as soon as the motor nerve is identified and slung in a vessel loop.

Neurovascular Anatomy

The latissimus dorsi, as the name implies, is the broadest muscle of the back, its superior fibers fanning out transversely across the angles of the scapula to reach the lumbodorsal fascia in the midline (superior margin) and anterolateral fibers descending vertically to the iliac crest. The tendon of latissimus dorsi joins the teres major and inserts into the medial aspect of the humerus as a conjoint tendon, forming the posterior axillary fold. The major vascular supply to latissimus dorsi arises from the subscapular–thoracodorsal axis (Fig. 17.1). The subscapular artery arises from the third part of the axillary artery, as it emerges under the pectoralis minor tendon. The subscapular artery soon sends off a large dorsal branch, the circumflex scapular artery, based on which the free fasciocutaneous scapula flap may be raised. Coursing beneath the subscapularis muscle, a large branch, the thoracodorsal artery, reaches the under surface of the latissimus dorsi, where it enters the fibers of the muscle accompanied by the thora-

Fig. 17.1 The vascular anatomical basis of the latissimus dorsi flap. Inset shows the consistent branching pattern of the subscapular vascular axis.

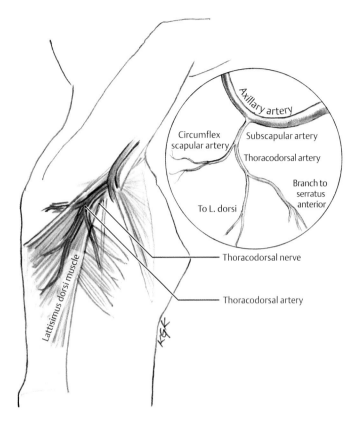

codorsal nerve. A branch of the thoracodorsal artery provides direct blood supply to the lower four slips of the serratus anterior muscle.

Thus the subscapular system offers multiple blocks of soft tissue and bone that may be transplanted based on a single vascular pedicle. Venous drainage is into the axillary vein through venae comitantes that accompany the thoracodorsal artery. Motor innervation of the latissimus dorsi muscle is via the thoracodorsal nerve, a branch of the posterior cord of the brachial plexus. The nerve accompanies the vascular pedicle and is found to enter the muscle approximately at the same point as the vessels. The nerve is also thought to offer proprioceptive innervation of the muscle. Experimental regeneration of sensory-to-motor nerve anastomoses in free muscle flaps has been documented, and clinical application of this phenomenon has reportedly enabled patients with foot reconstruction to "walk on" sensory-neurotized and restored deep proprioception of muscle flaps.[2]

The cutaneous territory of the latissimus dorsi musculocutaneous flap is very large; it overlies the central fibers of the muscle and overlaps with the territory of the serratus anterior muscle from the lateral aspect and with the territory of the scapular flap superiorly (**Fig. 17.2**).

Incisions and Dissection

The posterior axillary fold represented by the latissimus dorsi tendon is marked. This fold may be traced caudally along the lateral border of the muscle. The next key landmark is the angle of scapula, which is covered by transversely coursing fibers of the upper border of the latissimus dorsi muscle. The midline starting from the spinous process of T6 and running downward to the sacrum specifies the medial border of the muscle, whereas the inferior border is demarcated by the posterior portion of the superior iliac crest. A template of the defect to be reconstructed is drawn within the limits of these borders (**Fig. 17.3**). The skin island is cen-

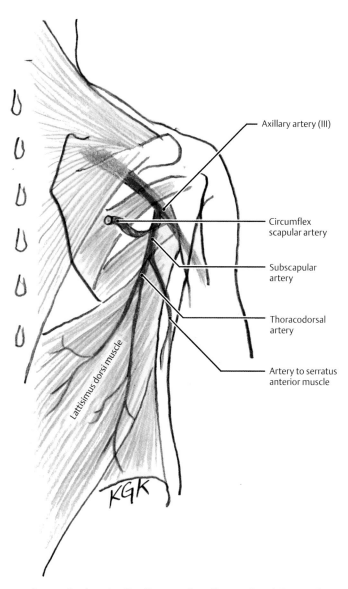

Fig. 17.2 The vascular anatomical basis of flaps based on the subscapular pool.

Axillary artery (III)

Circumflex scapular artery

Subscapular artery

Thoracodorsal artery

Artery to serratus anterior muscle

Lattisimus dorsi muscle

KGK

tered over the longitudinally coursing fibers of the latissimus dorsi muscle.

The initial approach to the neurovascular pedicle is identical to raising the serratus anterior flap: the anterior border of the cutaneous island is incised first, extending it as necessary in a lazy-S or zigzag pattern into the posterior axillary line. The lateral border of the latissimus dorsi muscle is retracted. The thoracodorsal neurovascular bundle is immediately visualized to be coursing beneath the muscle and can be traced caudally to enter the muscle substance

(**Fig. 17.4**). For the moment the pedicle is slung with a vessel loop. At this point muscle relaxing agents may be administered.

Now the posterior skin incision of the cutaneous island is completed and the muscle is divided as required, using monopolar cautery. As the vascular pedicle is followed centrally, one identifies the major branch to the serratus anterior muscle, and more proximally the circumflex scapular artery, which enters the triangular space dorsally. (Both of these may be sacrificed by division between ligating clips if an exceed-

Fig. 17.3 Planning of flaps based on the subscapular vascular axis. L., latissimus.

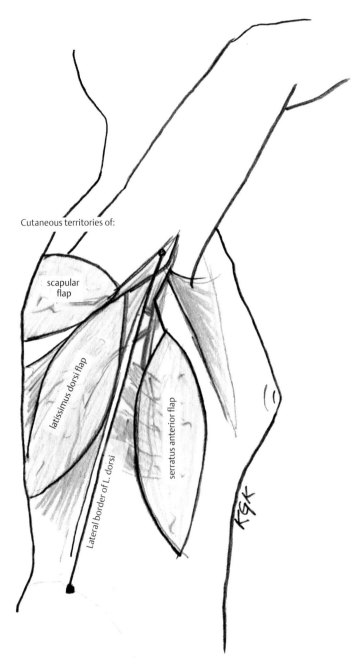

Cutaneous territories of:

scapular flap

latissimus dorsi flap

Lateral border of L. dorsi

serratus anterior flap

ingly long vascular pedicle of to the latissimus dorsi muscle flap is found necessary for meeting the demands of the recipient site.) Soon after, the tendon of the latissimus dorsi muscle is divided and the flap is isolated on its neurovascular bundle (**Fig. 17.5**). Now, low molecular weight dextran is administered to enhance microcirculation within the flap. As soon as the recipient site is ready for receiving the transfer, the vessels and nerve are divided between ligatures and the muscle is transferred. The muscle may be tailored as required based on its distinct intramuscular microvascular anatomy (**Fig. 17.6**).

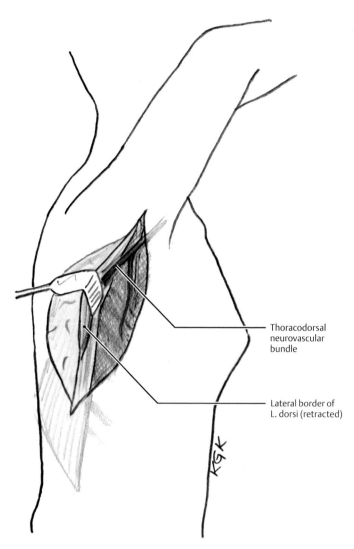

Fig. 17.4 Dissection of the latissimus (L.) dorsi flap.

Thoracodorsal
neurovascular
bundle

Lateral border of
L. dorsi (retracted)

Two large caliber suction drains are placed in the donor area. Usually wound closure is accomplished in layers by means of direct apposition of the skin borders after mobilizing them. Extensive skin harvest may rarely require grafting.

The vascular pedicle is usually approximately 10–15 cm in length, and may be lengthened further by sacrificing the branches and carrying the dissection up into the subscapular system. The vessels have diameters of ~2–3 mm.

Pitfalls

Latissimus dorsi is a reliable workhorse flap without known pitfalls. However, after harvesting large muscle portions, serous fluid may accumulate in the donor area. This is annoying, but usually subsides on repeated taps and compression dressings.

Fig. 17.5 Harvest and some variations of the latissimus dorsi flap.

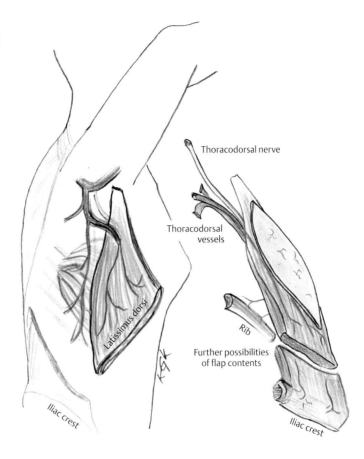

References

1 *Maxwell GP, Stueber K, Hoopes JE.* A free latissimus dorsi myocutaneous flap: case report. Plast Reconstr Surg 1978;62:462–466

2 *Chang KN, DeArmond SJ, Bunke HJ.* Sensory reinnervation in microsurgical reconstruction of the heel. Plast Reconstr Surg 1986; 78:652–664

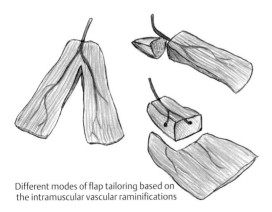

Different modes of flap tailoring based on the intramuscular vascular raminifications

Fig. 17.6 Some methods of debulking the latissimus dorsi flap based on its intrinsic vascular anatomy.

Chapter 18
The Scapular Skin Flap

The scapular cutaneous flap was one of the earliest free flaps to be clinically applied. The subscapular artery branches off the third part of the axillary artery, as we have already seen in the description of the latissimus dorsi and serratus anterior muscle flaps. It is one of the vessels with minimal, or practically no, variability of its consistent thoracodorsal and other arterial branches. Gilbert performed early cadaver dissections, isolating oblique skin territories based on the circumflex scapular arterial system, and later applied the knowledge clinically.[1] Others followed suit and delineated the characteristics of the cutaneous branches of the circumflex scapular artery more clearly, so that the territories of its two largest terminal branches were described.[2] This led to the formation of the transverse and oblique scapular cutaneous flaps, the latter also being called the "parascapular" flap. Further, other components, such as bone from the lateral border of the scapula[3] and deep fascia overlying the back muscles,[4] were added to the original cutaneous flap, making the scapular and parascapular flaps a more versatile option. Additionally, the scapular flaps offer the possibility of combining them with other muscular and bone flaps, all based on the subscapular vascular pool.

The scapular flap is a popular option among reconstructive surgeons, owing to its easy harvest, reliable and large caliber microvascular pedicle, as well as the availability of compound neighboring tissue blocks that may be raised with it.

Preparation

The scapular flap is advantageous for recipient defects located in the posterior parts of the body, since the patient is ideally placed in the prone position for the harvest of the scapular flap. This is also a disadvantage in reconstructing anteriorly located recipient sites, where patient repositioning will be necessary for scapular flap harvest. Thus in such situations, it appears logical, if possible, to choose other cutaneous flaps from the anterior body surface or the extremities. The vertically oriented scapular flap can also be raised with the patient in a lateral decubitus position. Preoperative Doppler examination of the triangular space will prove useful in locating the branches of the circumflex scapular vessels.

Neurovascular Anatomy

The harvestable cutaneous territory of the transverse scapular flap (~20 cm × 10 cm) is located between the angle and spine of the scapula, whereas the obliquely oriented parascapular flap (25 cm × 10 cm) is outlined, centered over the lateral border of the scapula. Both these territories are nourished by the two respective branches of the circumflex scapular artery that emerges to the suprafascial surface from the triangular space, bordered laterally by the long head of triceps and inferiorly by the teres major muscle belly and superiorly by the teres minor muscle (**Fig. 18.1**).

The triangular space should be included in the either of the above-mentioned flap geometries. The circumflex scapular artery may be traced to the subscapular artery, which in its turn arises from the third part of the axillary artery, lateral to the border of the subscapularis muscle. As the circumflex scapular artery curves around the lateral border of the scapula to "surface" through the triangular space, it gives off tiny branches to the teres major, teres minor, and infraspinatus muscles, as well as to the periosteal vessels of the scapular border, based on which a strip of bone may be raised with the flap. After emerging from the triangular space, the circumflex scapular artery takes a short caudal course (ca. 2–3 cm), after which it bifurcates into the transverse and vertical branches. Venous drainage of the flaps is through venae comitantes that accompany the arterial branches. Cutaneous nerves do not accompany the vessels. Sensory innervation of the flaps is achieved by segmental branches that run from medial to lateral and is usually

Fig. 18.1 The vascular anatomical basis of the scapular and parascapular flaps.

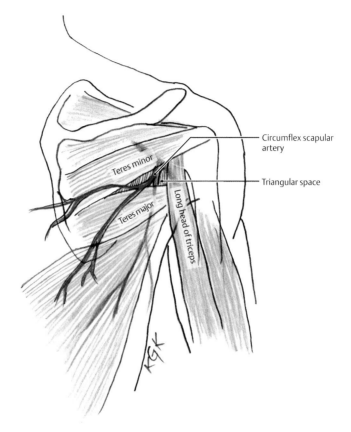

Fig. 18.2 Planning markings of the scapular and parascapular flaps.

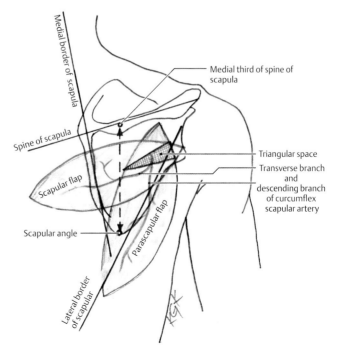

very tedious to trace. Thus the scapular flaps are mainly asensate.

Incisions and Dissection

The angle, spine, as well as the medial and lateral borders of the scapula can be well palpated and marked. The triangular space may be palpated as a depression slightly lateral to the point where the long head of triceps passes deep to the teres major muscle. This space is examined with a Doppler probe and marked. This point should be included in either of the flap configurations (**Fig. 18.2**). The transverse flap is drawn elliptically between the angle and spine of scapula measuring ~20 cm × 10 cm, which includes the triangular space. The verti-

cal flap will be centered on the lateral border of scapula.

The superior skin incision is placed first and dissection is performed in the depth into the triangular space. The vessels can be visualized here and are surrounded by globules of fat tissue (**Fig. 18.3**). Blunt separation is performed and the vessels are slung in a soft vessel loop. From then on, the dissection is straightforward: the rest of the marked skin incisions are completed and the flap is raised from medial to lateral (toward the isolated vascular pedicle) on a suprafascial plane. Care should be taken not to tug at the raised cutaneous flap (**Fig. 18.4**). The triangular space is opened with blunt retractors and the vascular pedicle is followed to its subscapular origin. The tiny perforating branches

Fig. 18.3   Dissection of the scapular flap.

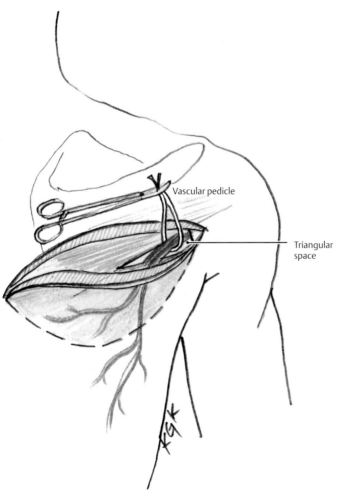

Vascular pedicle

Triangular space

Fig. 18.4 Harvest of the scapular flap.

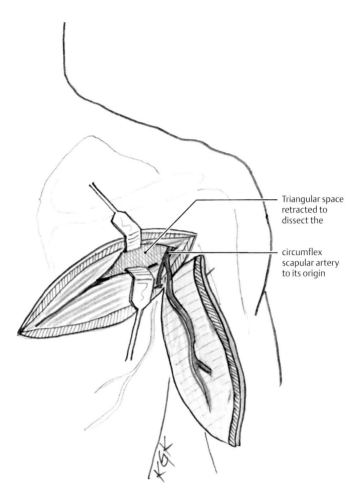

Triangular space retracted to dissect the

circumflex scapular artery to its origin

that supply the teres and infraspinatus muscles may be transected after bipolar cautery. As an alternative, thin cuffs of these muscles along with a strip of the lateral border of scapula may be raised with the flap (osteocutaneous flap). After tracing the circumflex scapular vessels to the subscapular system, the pedicle is transected between ligatures. Now the flap is ready to be transplanted. The microvessels of the pedicle are of the order of 1.5–3 mm in diameter; the pedicle length is ~6–8 cm when isolated at the triangular space. A suction Redon drain is placed in the wound after harvest. The skin borders are widely undermined, and primary wound closure is achieved in layers.

Pitfalls

Albeit a reliable and consistent cutaneous flap, requirements of patient repositioning during reconstruction of anteriorly located defects have made this flap less attractive, especially as other cutaneous flaps have been developed. However, this flap is far from being obsolete. Horizontal or vertical scarring on the scapular region after harvest can be annoying and cosmetically unpleasant, more so as the donor wound is closed under considerable tension. The other disadvantage of the flap is its asensate nature.

References

1 *Gilbert A, Teot L.* The free scapular flap. Plast Reconstr Surg 1982;69:601–604

2 *Nassif TM, Vidal L, Bovet JL, Bauder J.* The parascapular flap – A new cutaneous microsurgical free flap. Plast Reconstr Surg 1982;69:591–600

3 *Teot L, Souyris F, Bosse JP.* Pedicle scapular apophysis in congenital limb malformations. Ann Plast Surg 1992;29:332–340

4 *Kim PS, Gottlieb JR, Harris GD, Nagle DJ, Lewis VL.* The dorsal thoracic fascia: anatomic significance with clinical applications in reconstructive microsurgery. Plast Reconstr Surg 1987;79:72–80

Chapter 19
The Free Vascularized Rib Flap

The ribs, in particular the 7th through 9th, have three excellent interrelated sources of blood supply:[1] the proper nutrient artery,[2] the periosteal network arising from the segmental vessels, and[3] the perforating vessels from the muscular attachments, namely, from the serratus anterior and latissimus dorsi muscles. This enables harvest of the vascularized rib as a free flap in two different ways: either in compound form as an osteomuscular flap, based on the vascular pedicles of the muscle flaps, or as an osseous unit alone, based on the proper nutrient vessels.

Although there are reports on neo-functionally dependent post-transplantation hypertrophy of ribs used in lower extremities, the free rib flap has gained popularity mainly for reconstruction of the facial skeleton, especially of mandibular defects.[1–5] Vascularized bone tissue carries its own vascularity and is not dependent on the recipient bed, unlike free bone grafts; thus, such flaps are better suited for bone reconstruction in irradiated areas.[3–5] The rib flap can be combined with a cutaneous component overlying it, which will survive on the septal perforators, making it an interesting option for "monitoring" bone perfusion during the early, post-transfer phase. The harvest of a rib, or even two, leaves practically no deficits behind at the donor area, whereas free vascularized fibula may be considered a more privileged donor site. The choice of the flap, as we have already seen in other chapters, is dictated by the type of defect to be dealt with.

Preparation

A double lumen selective intubation of the bronchi is preferred. This way, the lung on the side of the operation may be temporarily deflated, so as to ease the rib harvest. (The rib is sometimes extremely adherent to the parietal pleura anteriorly, especially in the elderly, those with lung diseases, and smokers. When this phenomenon is encountered, the best way is to harvest a part of the parietal pleura with the rib.) The patient may be placed in the lateral or half-lateral position by raising the harvest side with a wedge cushion. The arm is abducted and placed in a hand rest.

Neurovascular Anatomy

The lower ribs, 7th through 9th, are best suited for harvest, since the neurovascular bundle is more easily identified in the lower ribs than in the upper ribs. These ribs receive their blood supply from two major sources: the intercostal segmental arteries originating from the thoracic aorta, which course into the intercostal spaces midway between the ribs; and the perforating arteries from the overlying latissimus dorsi and serratus anterior muscles. The rib flap raised is based on either of the two systems. The major branch of the intercostal artery arises from the aorta and reaches the intercostal groove lateral to the costal tubercle; it can be identified deep to the external and internal intercostal muscles on the posterior intercostal membrane (**Fig. 19.1**). Identifying this vessel at its origin is not required. Innervation is by means of the intercostal nerves that provide motor innervation of the intercostal muscles and sensory innervation to the skin overlying the rib. The intercostal nerves divide into posterior, lateral, and anterior sensory branches. The lateral branch accompanies the intercostal artery and vein. The entire rib can be harvested based on this bundle, which is located in the subcostal groove.

Incisions and Dissection

If an osteocutaneous flap is planned, the elliptical skin island should be marked overlying the lateral third of the 8th or 9th rib segment, where the ribs show a gentle curvature and can be easily palpated. Such planning includes the intercostal perforator in the skin island, which contains the sensory nerve that converts the skin island additionally into an innervated component. Large cutaneous perforators are located at the area of the anterior axillary line (**Fig. 19.2**).

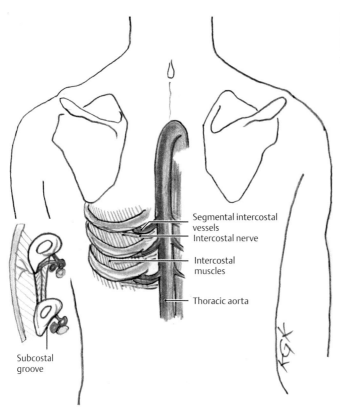

Fig. 19.1 The vascular anatomical basis of the vascularized rib flap. Inset: Sagittal view of the vascularity of the flap

Segmental intercostal vessels

Intercostal nerve

Intercostal muscles

Thoracic aorta

Subcostal groove

The upper border of the skin island is incised first and the dissection is carried into the depth reaching the intercostal space toward the intercostal muscles, carefully avoiding shearing the skin from the underlying rib due to overt retraction; rather, a cuff of muscle is left attached to preserve the vascularity of the skin island. Now the lower margin of the skin island is incised, and the dissection is carried into the depth reaching the intercostal muscles. The intercostal muscles are incised; no attempt is made to separate the parietal pleura from the inner surface of the rib. The lung on the side of harvest is deflated and one-lung respiration is performed to avoid injury to the visceral pleura or the lung itself. The parietal pleura underlying the rib is incised and will be raised later with the rib. As one incises the lower intercostal muscles, the vascular pedicle may be visualized to lie in the subcostal groove. It is a good policy to keep a muscle cuff attached to the inner surface of the rib, so as to prevent accidental injury to the vascular pedicle.

The anterior border of the planned bone flap is cut either with an oscillating saw, or with a Roos rib cutter (**Fig. 19.3**). The vessels are teased away from the subcostal groove at the area of the osteotomy and transected between ligating clips. Dissection is carried on to the posterior segment of the rib. Approximately 1–2 cm before the planned osteotomy, the neurovascular bundle is teased out of the inferior costal groove using a blunt nerve hook and slung with a vessel loop. Now the posterior osteotomy is completed whilst carefully avoiding tugging at the hanging rib segment. The neurovascular bundle is teased out of the posterior rib segment and left in situ as long as required. The neurovascular bundle is then ligated and transected. The length of the pedicle may be increased both by posterior mobilization and freeing the pedicle from the costal groove of the raised rib flap. The blood vessels arise posteriorly and reach the subcostal groove at the level of the costal tuberosity. It is seldom required to dissect the neurovascular pedicle more posteriorly, nor is this

Fig. 19.2 Planning markings for the harvest of the vascularized rib.

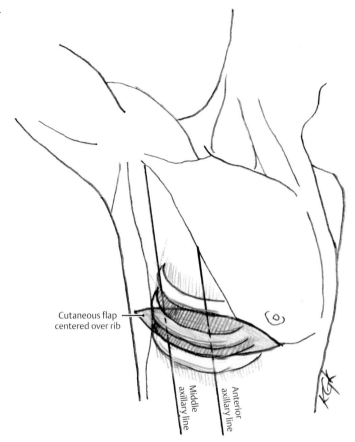

Cutaneous flap centered over rib

Middle axillary line

Anterior axillary line

warranted, because the vasculature to the spinal cord is located posterior to the costal tuberosity, and should not be jeopardized (**Fig. 19.4**).

Depending on the length of rib harvested, four to six circumferential sutures with #0 or #1 braided polyester suture material are placed around the rib above and below, but these are not yet tied. A rib approximator is used to pull these ribs above and below as near to each other as possible. Now the sutures are tied. A temporary chest tube is introduced into the pleural cavity and exteriorized through the skin above or below the skin incisions used for the harvest. Muscles overlying the defect are sutured in several layers. Then the lung is inflated and suction applied to the chest tube, which is removed soon after airtight closure has been achieved at the end of the skin sutures.

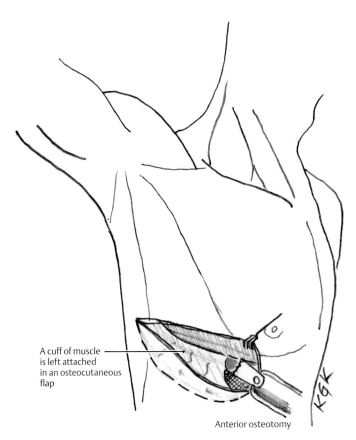

Fig. 19.3 Dissection of the vascularized rib flap.

A cuff of muscle is left attached in an osteocutaneous flap

Anterior osteotomy

Pitfalls

In comparison to other vascularized bone flaps, the rib is not a strong bone, which argues against its use in reconstruction of weightbearing areas. A nonvascularized rib transplant, such as used in calvarial or mandibular reconstruction, can rapidly revascularize at the recipient bed, particularly where the graft is split and there is a wide area of contact between the bone graft and the wound bed. Thus the free vascularized rib flap may be reserved for highly scarred and/or irradiated areas, where the vascularity has been compromised.

References

1 *Ostrup LT, Fredrickson JM*. Distant transfer of a free, living bone graft by microvascular anastomoses. An experimental study. Plast Reconstr Surg 1974;54:274–285

2 *Buncke HJ, Fumas DW, Gordon L, Achauer BM*. Free osteocutaneous flap from a rib to the tibia. Plast Reconstr Surg 1977;59:799–804

3 *Berggren A, Weiland AJ, Ostrup LT*. Bone scintigraphy in evaluating the viability of composite bone grafts revascularized by microvascular anastomoses, conventional autogenous bone grafts, and free non revascularized periosteal grafts. J Bone Joint Surg Am 1982; 64:799–809

Fig. 19.4 Harvest of the vascularized rib flap.

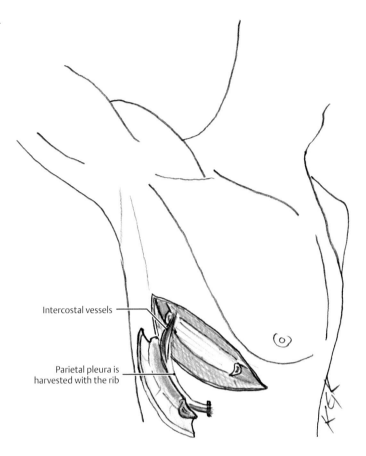

Intercostal vessels

Parietal pleura is harvested with the rib

4 *Berggren A, Weiland AJ, Dorfman H.* Free vascularized bone grafts: Factors affecting their survival and ability to heal the recipient bone defects. Plast Reconstr Surg 1982;69:19–29

5 *Ostrup LT, Tam CS.* Bone formation in a free, living bone graft transferred by microvascular anastomoses. A quantitative microscopic study using fluorochrome markers. Scand J Plast Reconstr Surg 1975;9:101–106

Chapter 20
The Free Greater Omentum Flap

The greater omentum is an apron of richly vas-cularized fat tissue guarding the abdominal cavity. The right and left gastroepiploic vessels form a rich vascular network among the layers of the omentum, which is additionally interwo-ven with a rich lymphatic network, qualifying its use for cases of lymphedema of the extremi-ties, for example, after axillary or inguinal dis-section. The greater omentum flap is further utilized in avascular situations, such as ische-mic statuses of lower extremities, sequelae of radiation therapy and burns, as well as revascu-larization of the ischemic heart and brain.[1] Due to the thin layer of fat tissue, a segment of vas-cularized omentum may be used to restore slid-ing planes, such as those found around scarred joints and tendons.

The first successful experimental and clinical free vascularized transfer of the greater omen-tum was performed by Bunke and McLean.[2] The greater omentum flap is reliable, having a con-stant vascular anatomy. As is also the case with other anterior donor sites, a two-team ap-proach is possible in reconstructing defects of the anterior or lateral body parts.

Preparation

Previous abdominal surgery might jeopardize the harvest of the entire greater omentum. However, depending on the type of previous abdominal surgery, parts of the omentum might still be available. The patient is placed in the supine position. As one team performs the midline laparotomy, the other team prepares the recipient site.

Vascular Anatomy

The greater omentum may be compared to a double-layered curtain, one layer attached to the transverse colon and the other to the greater curvature of the stomach, hanging

down and covering the contents of the abdomi-nal cavity. The rich vasculature is formed by the anastomoses between the left and right gastro-epiploic arteries entering the greater omentum from the respective ends of the greater gastric curvature (Fig. 20.1). This vascular network also provides multiple branches to the celiac struc-tures to which the greater omentum is at-tached, namely, the greater curvature of the stomach and the transverse colon. Venous drainage is through comitant veins that accom-pany the respective left and right gastroepiploic arteries. The length of the vascular pedicle is of no concern, since it can be elongated as re-quired by mobilizing the vascular network be-tween the left and right pedicles.

Flap harvest is usually based on the right gastroepiploic vessels, since these are some-what larger than the left. However, mobiliza-tion based on the left-sided vessels is also pos-sible, for instance, in pedicled greater omentum flap used in mediastinal wound coverage.

Incisions and Dissection

Harvesting of the greater omentum as a free flap is quite straightforward. As one team works at the recipient site, debriding the wound and dissecting the donor vessels for anastomoses, the other team simultaneously harvests the greater omentum. Laparotomy is done either via an upper midline incision or a transverse in-cision in the upper epigastric quadrant. As the abdominal cavity is opened, the greater omen-tum is seen immediately under the peritoneum. The omentum is carefully separated from its at-tachments to both the transverse colon and the greater curvature of the stomach, ligating the multiple gastroepiploic vessels and collateral branches to the stomach and transverse colon. The right gastroepiploic vascular pedicle is identified at the gastroduodenal junction; a segment of these vessels (its length depending on the requisites of the recipient site) is care-fully denuded under optical binocular loupe magnification. As soon as the recipient site is ready to receive the transplant, the vascular pedicle of the flap is divided between ligatures and the omentum transferred (Fig. 20.2). If the goal of transferring the greater omentum is to

Fig. 20.1 The vascular anatomical basis of the greater omentum flap.

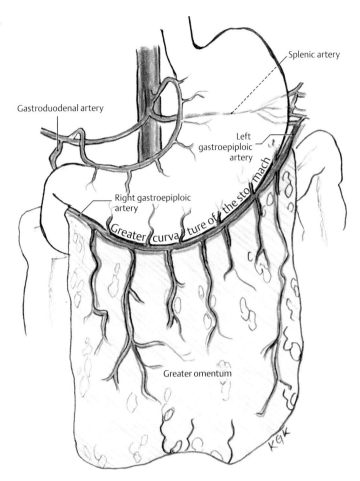

Splenic artery

Gastroduodenal artery

Left gastroepiploic artery

Right gastroepiploic artery

Greater curvature of the stomach

Greater omentum

enhance or even re-establish lymphatic drainage, then the enlarged lymphatic vessels at the recipient area are anastomosed to the venous network of the omentum in an end-to-side fashion.

Perioperative administration of antibiotics is deemed necessary in omental flaps, since fat tissue has a tendency to rapidly conduce infection. This is especially true in nonvascularized fat tissue; thus, it is also recommended to administer low molecular weight dextran in a tapering scheme for 5 days after surgery to preserve and enhance flap microcirculation, as well as heparinize the patient for 5 days. This is controlled by prolonging the partial thromboplastin time to the double of its preoperative value; usually the target value for heparinization in adults is 60 seconds.

Pitfalls

There are no major pitfalls involved in harvesting the free greater omentum flap. However, with the availability of many new muscle and myocutaneous free flaps, omental transplantation is becoming obsolete. It appears sensible to choose one of the more accessible muscle transplants for tackling difficult wound closure problems and avoid the risks connected with laparotomy. Previous abdominal surgery also eliminates the omentum as a free transplant, since the greater omentum, also colloquially called the "policeman of the abdominal cavity" approaches an inflamed area and scars with it in the process of healing.

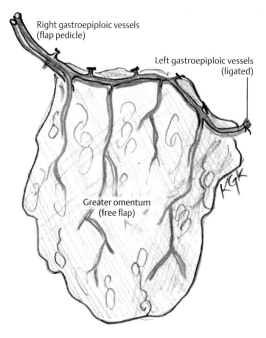

Right gastroepiploic vessels
(flap pedicle)

Left gastroepiploic vessels
(ligated)

Greater omentum
(free flap)

Fig. 20.2   The harvested greater omentum flap.

References

1 *Nikonenko AS, Pertsov VI, Osaulenko VV, Ermolaev EV, Ksenzov AY.* Technical aspects of revascularizing transplantation of omentum majus on myocardium, upper extremity and brain. Klin Khir 2000;8:23–26

2 *McLean DH, Buncke HJ* Jr. Autotransplant of omentum to a large scalp defect, with microsurgical revascularization. Plast Reconstr Surg 1972;49:268–274

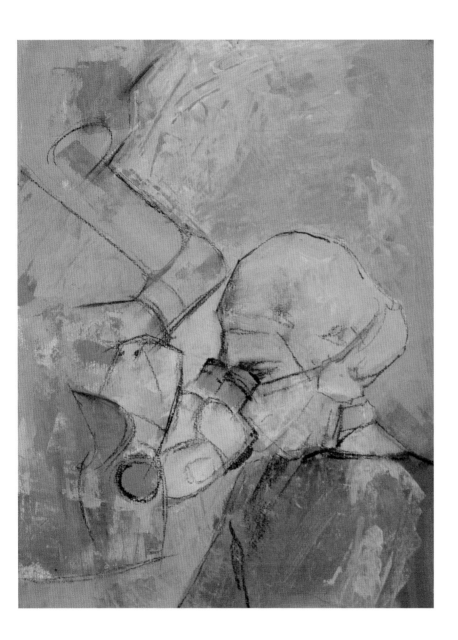

Part 4
Appendices

Part 4
Appendices

The goal of a reconstructive microsurgeon in the management of tissue defects is to obtain a closed, stable wound as soon as possible. In this task the surgeon preserves as much undamaged tissue as possible, avoids infectious complications, and attempts to limit the amount of scar formation. The method of wound closure will depend on the location, mechanism and extent of injury, and the degree of contamination. The techniques of wound closure range from simple, primary suturing of the wound edges to free tissue transplantation using microsurgical techniques after preparing the wound bed for flap reception. Optimal management of wound defects demands a thorough knowledge and understanding of the fundamental concepts influencing the process of wound healing.

Wound healing is a topic in its own right, which has been dealt with in several published volumes, and its inclusion in a manual such as this on flap raising techniques appears a little far-fetched. However, in the following chapters, I have attempted to treat comprehensively three basic topics of paramount importance for the successful implementation of microvascular flaps: (a) general understanding of microvascular anatomy and patterns of vasculature of soft tissue flaps; (b) microsurgical instrumentation and modes of optical magnification; and (c) microvascular and microneural suturing techniques.

It is important to keep microsurgical skills well honed by constant practice. A few "kitchen exercises" of microsurgical suturing techniques are included in the following chapters. The reader might favorably profit from some of these tips, since they have helped me to keep my surgical techniques well polished during periods of clinical inactivity.

Chapter 21
Vascular Patterns of Soft-Tissue Flaps

Flaps are blocks of tissue that can be isolated on their nourishing vascular pedicle and transplanted elsewhere on the body to replenish tissue deficiencies. More precisely, flaps are indicated for covering wound beds, where the exposed structures are devoid of capillary circulation on their surfaces. The discovery and delineation of the microcirculatory anatomy of soft-tissue structures have revolutionized the concepts and application of flaps for wound management.

The Vascular Pattern of the Skin

Contemporary knowledge of the microcirculation of the skin holds that the skin is supplied by dermal and subdermal plexuses of microvessels. These plexuses receive significant contributions from vertically oriented perforators of relatively large vessels located in the underlying muscles or fascia, which may be isolated under loupe magnification (**Fig. 21.1**). The muscles and/or fascia are, in turn, nourished by one or more, relatively larger vascular pedicles. In a few areas of the body surface, the skin is supplied directly by reliably large, direct cutaneous arteries that run in the subcutaneous fat tissue.

Based upon their microvascular anatomy, cutaneous flaps may be classified as random or axial pattern flaps, which are located adjacent to the defect (local flaps). Tissue blocks that are remote to the defect and need transplantation based on their vascular pedicles are termed distant flaps.

Historically, before the vascular patterns of the skin were delineated, cutaneous flaps were designed according to geometric principles, without taking the underlying nourishing circulation into consideration. These "random" pattern flaps were based only on the dermal and subdermal plexuses, and the vertically oriented perforators from the underlying muscle and/or fascial layers became severed, since the flaps were raised on a subcutaneous plane (**Fig. 21.2**). Thus such flaps survived only on indulging in a flap geometry that matched the length and width; certain richly vascularized areas such as the facial and scalp skin being exceptions, where the length of the random pattern flap may be safely increased. Failure to abide by this geometrical pattern runs the risk of partial necrosis of random pattern flaps.

Contrary to random pattern flaps, axial pattern flaps are designed to include a large vascular pedicle that is known to reliably supply the overlying flap (**Fig. 21.3**). These axial vessels may be located in any of the underlying

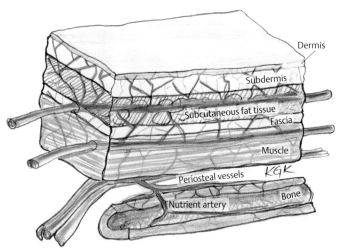

Fig. 21.1 The microvascular anatomical basis of vascularized flaps.

Dermis

Subdermis

Subcutaneous fat tissue

Fascia

Muscle

Periosteal vessels

Nutrient artery

Bone

KGK

Fig. 21.2 The geometrical design of a random pattern skin flap.

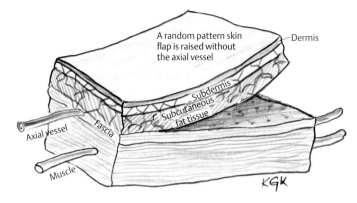

Fig. 21.3 The geometrical design of an axial pattern skin flap.

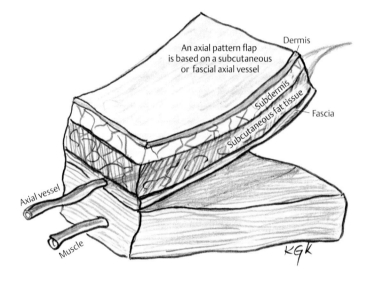

layers: subcutaneous, fascial, or muscle. Salient examples of axial pattern cutaneous flaps are the groin flap based on the superficial circumflex iliac artery that runs through the subcutaneous tissue, and the forehead flap for nose reconstruction. As long as the axial nourishing vessels are included, the flaps may be raised without regard to their geometrical pattern or length-to-width ratio. As per this description, any flap with an individual vascular supply comes under the category of axial pattern flaps. An axial pattern flap may preserve its proximal tissue connection and be advanced or rotated (local rotational / advancement flap); the flap may be dissected circumferentially, left connected to the body only on the axial vessels and

moved to an adjacent part of the given body region (regional flap), or a flap may be completely isolated based on its axial pedicle and transected from the body to be transplanted elsewhere (free flap).

The Vascular Pattern of the Muscles

Delineation of vascular supply to muscles both in the lab and clinic in the 1970s has revolutionized plastic surgery.[1–4] Based on the anatomical knowledge of the location of the vascular supply, practically any muscle in the body may be mobilized and transferred to neighboring regions. As already mentioned, all superficially located muscles supply the overlying skin by means of the vertical musculocutaneous perforators (**Fig. 21.1**). Thus the harvest of any superficial muscle may be combined with the overlying skin to form a musculocutaneous flap. However, in a musculocutaneous flap the presence of subcutaneous adipose tissue between the skin and the muscle flap causes shearing movements, which is undesired in reconstructing certain areas, for example, the sole of the foot, hand, or scalp. Thus in such situations the bare muscle is transplanted to provide a richly vascularized bed upon which a split-thickness mesh graft may be placed.

The potential usefulness of a muscle is determined by its pattern of blood supply. The vascular anatomy of muscles has been delineated as to the size, number, and location of the vascular pedicles. Accordingly, Mathes and Nahai classified vascular patterns of muscles into five types as follows[5]:

A *Mathes and Nahai type 1* muscle has one vascular pedicle (**Fig. 21.4**). The gastrocnemius (considered separately as the medial and lateral heads), tensor fasciae latae, and rectus femoris muscles are some examples of this type that consistently have only one vascular pedicle. Blocks of these muscles together with huge areas of overlying skin can be transferred on their pedicles.

A *Mathes and Nahai type 2* muscle has one or more dominant vascular pedicles located at the origin of the muscle and several smaller secondary vascular pedicles entering the belly of the muscle along its course (**Fig. 21.5**). The gracilis muscle falls into this category. As a rule, the multiple vascular pedicles form a plexus within the muscle. Thus the revascularization of the dominant vascular pedicle is usually sufficient to guarantee survival of the entire muscle at the recipient site.

A *Mathes and Nahai type 3* muscle has two large (both dominant) vascular pedicles, each arising from a separate regional vessel and anastomosing inside the matter of the muscle (**Fig. 21.6**). Rectus abdominis, gluteus maximus, and serratus anterior muscles are examples of this type. Each pedicle has an equal share of the vascular supply, however the territories overlap. Revas-

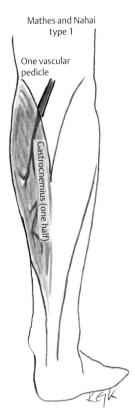

Fig. 21.4 Classification of muscle vascularity: type 1.

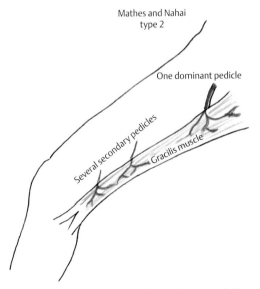

Fig. 21.5 Classification of muscle vascularity: type 2.

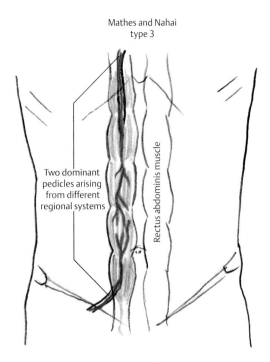

Fig. 21.6 Classification of muscle vascularity: type 3.

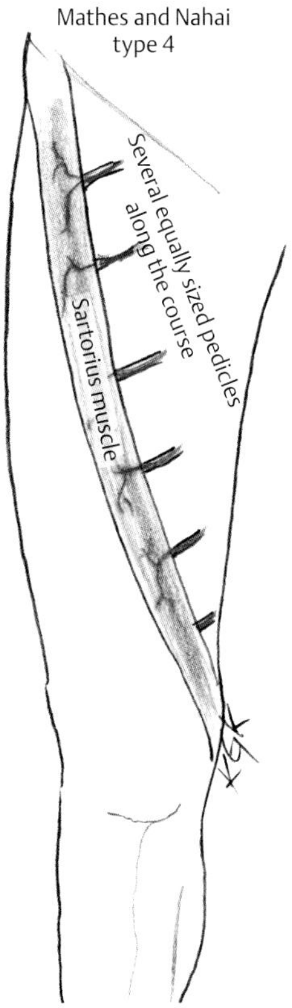

Fig. 21.7 Classification of muscle vascularity: type 4.

cularization of one pedicle at the recipient site ensures survival of the whole muscle block.

A *Mathes and Nahai type 4* muscle is supplied by several equally sized vascular pedicles that enter the muscle along its entire course (**Fig. 21.7**). The vascular territories, although they overlap each other and are in a position to take over a neighboring territory, when consecutively ligated will not be able to take over distantly located territories. This is a principal difference to the type-2 blood supply, where one dominant pedicle will take over the entire circulation of the muscle. Thus the type 4 muscle is not an attractive option for transferring whole muscles. In this case, either only parts of the muscle are used or multiple vascular pedicles require reconnection at the recipient site.

A *Mathes and Nahai type 5* muscle has one major vascular pedicle entering at the site of its insertion and is additionally nourished by multiple segmentlike vessels of lesser caliber (**Fig. 21.8**). Latissimus dorsi and pectoralis major are the only two muscles that come under this category. These muscles can be mobilized and rotated to a defect on a given region based on either of the vascular pedicles.

The Mathes and Nahai classification of muscle flaps is based on the vascular pattern and helps predict the reliability of a particular muscle, its arc of rotation, and availability for free transfer. Accordingly, type 1 and type 5 muscles are quite reliable for free transfer; type 2 and type 3 muscles, although reliable, are not usually preferred, whereas the utility of a type 4 muscle is strictly limited.

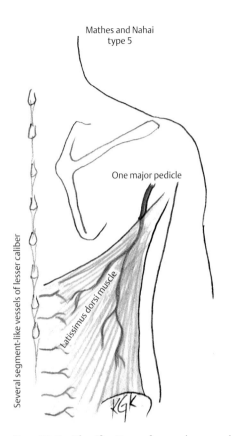

Fig. 21.8 Classification of muscle vascularity: type 5.

References

1 Mathes SJ, Nahai F. *Clinical Application for Muscle and Musculocutaneous Flaps.* St. Louis, Mo: Mosby; 1979.
2 *Mathes SJ, Vasconez LO, Jurkiewicz MJ.* Extensions and further applications of muscle flap transposition. Plast Reconstr Surg 1977;60: 6–10
3 *McCraw JB, Dibbell DG.* Experimental definition of independent myocutaneous vascular territories. Plast Reconstr Surg 1977;60:212–220
4 *McCraw JB, Dibbell DG, Carraway JH.* Clinical definition of independent myocutaneous vascular territories. Plast Reconstr Surg 1977;60:341–352
5 *Mathes SJ, Nahai F.* Classification of the vascular anatomy of muscles: experimental and clinical correlation. Plast Reconstr Surg 1981;67:177–187

Chapter 22
Instrumentation for Microsurgery

Flap surgery is a discipline that requires compe-
tence in the surgical manipulation of tissues,
skills that lie at opposite ends of a scale from
microsurgery to macrosurgery. Just as the flap
surgeon needs to master bone manipulation,
handling of high speed saws, drills, burrs,
plates, wires, screws, so he or she should excel
in microminiature manipulation of the most
delicate vessels and nerves under high optical
magnification. Two interrelated areas of modern industry have served to revolutionize surgical practice in the last five decades, without
which flap surgery would not have been possible: (a) optical magnification, and (b) the
manufacture of microscopic suture material.
Fine-tipped instruments for manipulating the
microstructures and sutures were adopted from
watchmakers and jewelers and brought into
surgical practice much earlier than microsuture
manufacture.

Optical Magnification

Optical magnification used in surgery has undergone an entire process of evolution, starting
with the simple biconvex lens and ending with
the contemporary operating microscope. Today's operating microscope, shown schemati-
cally in **Fig. 22.1**, is the result of a fascinating
mix of achievements and advances in optics,
light physics, fiber optics, mechanical engineer-
ing, electronics, computing sciences, and robot-
ics. Rotational characteristics of the microscope
have enabled the precise focussing and crystal
clear beaming of anatomical structures located
in the most remote corners of the body; various
aspects of the clivus and the pituitary fossa are
examples (**Fig. 22.2**). By pressing a button with
a finger tip, or even by clenching a mouthpiece
between the teeth while the hands are still at
work, the surgeon is able to trigger intricate
electronic mechanisms that move an operating
microscope weighing approximately two tons

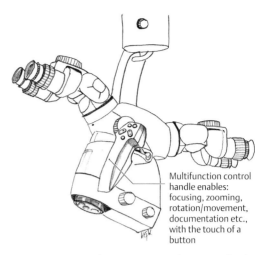

Multifunction control
handle enables:
focusing, zooming,
rotation/movement,
documentation etc.,
with the touch of a
button

Fig. 22.1 A schematic reproduction of the
modern-day operating microscope.

to suit the position of his or her head with respect to the anatomical structures being manipulated. Electronically activated anatomical
navigation that is based on preoperative diag-
nostic images, in particular neuronavigation,
are fused with the live stream, three-
dimensional microscopic images during surgery to enhance precision in the tracking of
specific anatomical structures.

As is evident here, the effective utilization of
an operating microscope requires, as does en-
doscopic surgery, the training and practice of
efficient hand–eye coordination. This skill can
be developed by no other means than directly
using the technology. It is to be anticipated that
the higher the power of magnification is, the
slower the movements of the surgeon. Wanting
to be "quick" in such a situation, as I observed
during my learning curve, only makes things
worse and one ends up with a lengthy and com-
plicated procedure. Phases of microsurgical
manipulations during a surgical operation
should show a steady and assured pace from
beginning to end, climaxing in an uncomplicated and successful achievement of the
planned phase. Furthermore, it is wise to bring
in the microscope comfortably in advance
before dire necessity demands it—better than
to struggle with microscopic structures under
the low magnification offered by binocular
loupes.

Fig. 22.2 Rotation and mobility of the operating microscope.

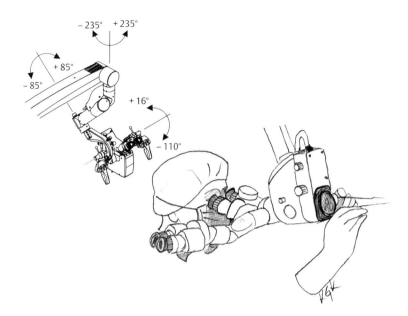

Operating microscopes come in two categories: ceiling mounted or floor mounted. A ceiling mounted microscope spares useful space in a modern operating room that harbors other technologies; the disadvantages are that the microscope cannot be moved to another room and cannot be stored off-site, thus will be found occupying space in other procedures where its use is not called for. The floor-mounted microscope occupies valuable operating room space; however, it can be moved to other rooms for usage. I have found it advantageous to use binocular Galilean loupes of 2.5× magnification starting from the first skin incision, till the period when higher magnification is demanded, and then afterward for completing the procedure till the end of wound closure (**Fig. 22.3**). One might argue with this practice; however, this small magnification ensures precision in macrosurgical manipulations, for example, identification of small perforators, precise bipolar cautery of bleeders, macrosurgical suture placement, etc., which in the end, surprisingly, saves a considerable amount of operating time. Additionally, I also have a pair of custom-made 8.0× prismatic magnifying loupes in my possession; these I use while operating in rooms other than ours, where a surgical microscope will not be available at short notice (**Fig. 22.4**).

It is a false impression of nonusers that wearing loupes will be tiring during long procedures. On the contrary, as one gets used to the proper use of surgical telescopic loupes, something appears to be missing when operating without them!

Microsutures

Synthetic threads of diameters ranging from 200 μm (8–0 suture) to 50 μm (12–0 suture) are used to perform anastomoses or sutures of microvessels and nerves. The needles are fabri-

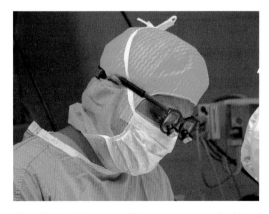

Fig. 22.3 2.5× magnifying custom-made binocular surgical loupes.

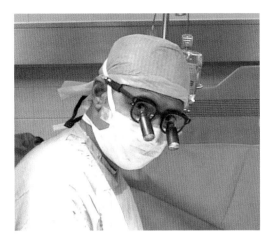

Fig. 22.4 8.0× magnifying custom-made binocular surgical loupes.

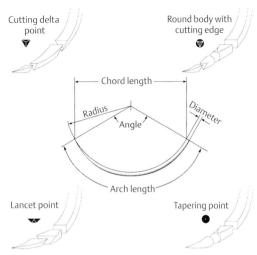

Fig. 22.5 Some physical characteristics of microsurgical needles.

cated of hardened steel, and are precision pointed and honed under a microforge. Microforging allows an ideal diameter ratio between the needle and suture minimizing, even eliminating, the jump at the needle–suture junction. The ideal needle will be stiff enough to offer resistance during penetration of different types of tissues (e.g., slippery vs hardened vessels), appropriately flat-pressed at the holding point to offer stability in the needle driver and side-pressed to enable bending resistance. Several specialized needle tips are manufactured for the penetration of different tissue types: vascular taper point, taper cutting, delta point and lancet point are some examples (**Fig. 22.5**).

Microsurgical Instruments

There are a quite a few commercial catalogues dedicated to microsurgical instruments alone. However, one needs no more than three of four of them during an entire procedure. Keeping the numbers small, but essential, additionally makes communication with the scrubbed nurse easy and quick. Microsurgical instruments (excluding those used in emergency procedures) are like fountain pens—they should be surgeon-specific. Instruments should not be too light or too heavy—they should be heavy enough to sit comfortably between the fingers in a pinch grip, and light enough to be rotated and manip-

ulated easily with the fingertips. The length of the instruments depends on the specific demands of the surgery, ranging from microvas-

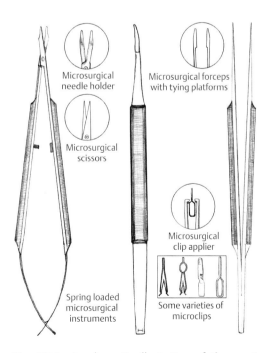

Fig. 22.6 A schematic illustration of the most useful microsurgical instruments.

cular anastomoses at the base of the skull requiring long, bayonet-shaped instruments, to short, straight ones used in hand surgical procedures.

For performing a microanastomosis, the scrub nurse's active table should contain—apart from the minimal amount of macroinstruments found in active use—one microneedle driver, two microforceps, one pair of microscissors, and one clip applier (**Fig. 22.6**). The side table should contain one more set of these, and additionally, several microvascular clips and microvessel and nerve approximators. Sutures ranging from 8–0 to 11–0 should be available in the operating room in readiness to be opened immediately as required.

Chapter 23
Microvascular Anastomoses and Microneural Sutures

The performance of microsutures, as already mentioned, requires excellent hand–eye coordination, skills that can be achieved by consistent training and constant practice. The phenomenon of hand dominance should ideally almost disappear while working under an operating microscope—one should be able to perform fine motor movements with both hands alike. The beginner may want to hone the skills of his or her nondominant hand through simple, but meaningful, exercises such as throwing a basketball, using keys to open locks, dialing numbers into a cellular phone—all with the nondominant hand. Training the nondominant hand also automatically trains the dominant one. In most situations of microsurgical manipulation, the elbow or the wrists are supported by a rest. Supporting the elbows or the wrists reduces physiological tremor during microsurgical work. However, certain circumstances, such as working in the depth or remote corners, warrant free-hand working without support. One should be prepared for this, and simulate such situations in experiments. Although microsurgical manipulations foresee nothing but fine motor functions of the hand and rarely the forearms, honed shoulder and arm muscles are also prerequisites. Holding the forearm and hand in unsupported constant positions in space requires fine-tuning of the large muscles of the arms and shoulders.

Handling Microsurgical Instruments

Microsurgical instruments are held in a pinch grip between the index finger and the thumb, the middle and ring fingers supporting the instrument from underneath (**Fig. 23.1**). The tip of the instrument is turned or rotated as required by slight pill-rolling movements between the index finger and the thumb. The ranges of movement at the metacarpophalangeal and interphalangeal joints are utilized to advance or

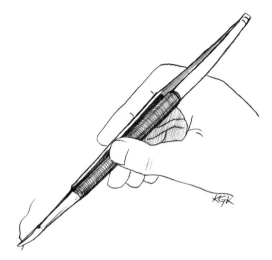

Fig. 23.1 A microsurgical instrument is held like a fountain pen.

retract the tip of the instrument. In situations where support of the wrists or elbows is not available, an outstretched little finger serves to minimize physiological hand tremor (**Fig. 23.2**).

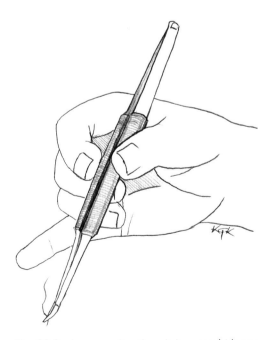

Fig. 23.2 In some situations it is a good idea to extend the little finger to support the hand.

Preparing a Microvessel for Anastomosis

The microvessels of the flaps, as they are cut during harvest, are not suitable for anastomoses. They have to be freed from loose connective tissue adherent to the adventitia for a distance of 2–8 mm from the end. Failure to do this runs the risk of the connective tissue accidentally getting entrapped into the vessel lumen, predisposing thrombotic complications. A quick and effective way to remove the connective tissue is to grasp it and pull it across the vessel end, which can now be seen under the translucent tissue. Then the connective tissue is cut in one sweep, taking care not to cut the vessel itself. The remaining tissue retracts itself, freeing the vessel end for anastomosis (**Fig. 23.3**). This manipulation is also termed "circumcision" of the vessel in colloquial surgical language. After that, the vessel is thoroughly flushed with heparinized solution.

The Microvascular Suture

Caution should be exercised when grasping the vessel wall between the branches of the forceps so as no to crush the intimal layer. The vessel is rather held by its adventitial outer layer. For making the suture from outside to inside, both the branches of the polished and blunt microforceps are introduced into the lumen, separating the back wall from the front. Then the needle is driven through the wall. For driving the needle from inside to outside, the adventitial layer of the vessel end is grasped with the forceps and the front wall of the vessel is lifted off the back. Then the needle is driven from inside to out (**Fig. 23.4**).

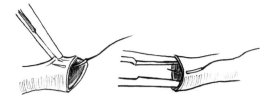

Fig. 23.4 Techniques of the first bite in a microvascular anastomosis.

Tying a Microsurgical Knot

This is done exclusively with instruments. With the needle holder in the dominant hand and the forceps in the other, the suture of the opposite end is grasped with the needle holder. The suture is then looped twice around the forceps, after which the other suture end is grasped with the forceps. Pulling the instruments apart throws the double reef knot (**Fig. 23.5**). The knot should be thrown without a kink. Usually not more than three knots are required to offer suture stability; I find a 2–1-1 knot pattern adequate for this purpose.

Microvascular Anastomosis

Several types of microvascular anastomoses need to be mastered: end-to-end, end-to-side, side-to-side, and finally the confluence anastomosis, where two vessel lumens are connected end-to-side in one anastomosis (**Fig. 23.6**). It is important to choose an appropriate suture material: too large a suture will make a clumsy

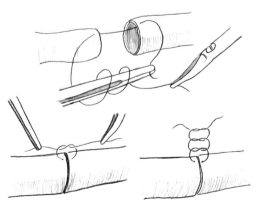

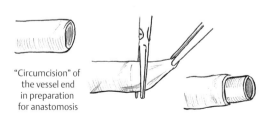

"Circumcision" of the vessel end in preparation for anastomosis

Fig. 23.3 Preparation of a vessel end for microvascular anastomosis.

Fig. 23.5 Technique of throwing knots with microinstruments.

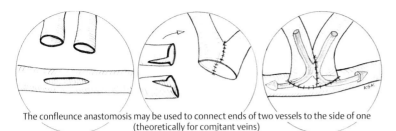

Fig. 23.6 A schematic representation of the steps in a confluence microvascular anastomosis.

The confleunce anastomosis may be used to connect ends of two vessels to the side of one (theoretically for comitant veins)

anastomosis, which might get blocked; too fine a suture will mandate the placement of many sutures, predispose leakage, and eventually the anastomosis might also get blocked. An ideal anastomosis is completed on first intension, with no need for secondary corrections or leaking areas.

In performing an end-to-end anastomosis, the corner sutures are made first, followed by the suture of the front wall facing the surgeon. Thenceforth the vessel is turned around 180°, along with the clips; the front wall sutures are examined through the lumen for adequacy and the back wall sutures are completed. Usually eight sutures suffice for a vessel ranging from 1–1.5 mm to achieve a hermetic anastomosis (**Fig. 23.7**).

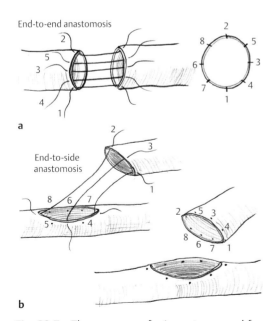

Fig. 23.7 The sequence of microsutures used for a microvascular anastomosis.

In performing anastomosis of a vessel end-to-side, the slit on the side of the vessel is made one and a half times larger than the diameter of the vessel to be connected. The end vessel is cut obliquely to increase its luminal diameter. The first suture is at the heel of the end vessel, followed by the one at the toe. If the side vessel can be rotated (this is not possible at some locations of the skull base), the front wall sutures are completed. Then the vessel is turned and the back wall is completed, after scrutinizing the sutures of the front wall through the semi-open lumen (**Fig. 23.7**). If, as mentioned above, the vessel cannot be rotated, then the back wall is sutured first in a continuous suture through the lumen of the vessel first. Then the front wall is undertaken. Usually 8 to 12 sutures are required for an end-to-side anastomosis of a vessel with a diameter measuring 1–1.5 mm.

Microneural Suture

Microsurgical suture of nerves should ensure adequate epineural closure of fascicles, so that neuromas in continuity caused by fascicles growing astray are avoided. Thus, the microsuture should pass through both the epineurium and the fascicle located in the periphery of both sides (**Fig. 23.8**). I would not advocate an interfascicular connection in suturing a compound nerve, since this only increases the amount of foreign material inside a nerve. The sutures are kept to the minimum; the rest of the connection being completed with fibrin glue. After placing the sutures, fibrin glue is applied circumferentially around the anastomosis; any excess glue is immediately sucked off, so as to prevent clumping. As a result, the anastomosis site will be wrapped in a thin, translucent layer of fibrin glue. Usually three or four sutures,

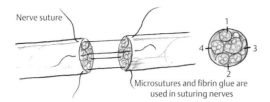

Fig. 23.8 Technique and sequence of microsutures in connecting micronerves.

combined with fibrin glue are quite adequate to connect nerves of diameters ranging from 1 to 4 mm.

Kitchen Exercises

Microanastomoses require constant practice, as do flap raising techniques. In an ideal situation, the clinician should nurture constant contact with the anatomy and animal experimentation laboratories. This requires an infrastructure, which is not always provided, especially in non-teaching centers. However, microsurgical skills can still be kept honed by some kitchen exercises. Many models have been proposed to this effect. I found the biological model proposed by Hino et al.[1] to be the most appropriate. They extract microvessels running through the inner aspect of fresh chicken wings, which may be obtained cheaply at any supermarket, and use them for training in anastomosis techniques (**Fig. 23.9**). I modified this idea a little by mounting an explanted vessel on a stand.[2]

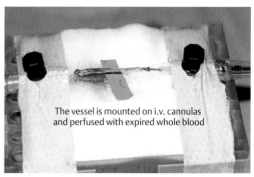

Fig. 23.10 Mounting and perfusion of a microvessel for simulation of a live model.

Either end of the explanted vessel was connected to intravenous catheters and expired; packed red blood cell concentrates or whole blood obtained from the blood bank was circulated through this microvascular system (**Fig. 23.10**). Thus a real situation was simulated in the experiment.

It needs to be mentioned and stressed again that it is a prudent idea to simulate difficult situations in experiments, such as creating high troughs to enhance depth of the structures manipulated, wearing out-sized gloves, and operating without hand-rests.

References

1 *Hino A.* Training in microsurgery using a chicken wing artery. Neurosurgery 2003; 52:1495–1498
2 *Krishnan KG, Dramm P, Schackert G.* A simple and viable in vitro perfusion model for training microvascular anastomoses. Microsurgery 2004;24:335–338

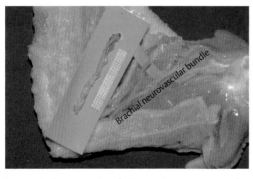

Fig. 23.9 Harvest of the microneurovascular bundle from the chicken wing for training purposes.

Index